Advances in Drug Research

Volume 10

Advances in Drug Research

Series Editors

N. J. HARPER

Sterling Winthrop, Research and Development
Newcastle upon Tyne, England

and

ALMA B. SIMMONDS

Chelsea College
University of London, England

Volume 10

edited by Alma B. Simmonds

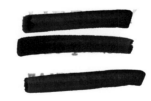

1975

ACADEMIC PRESS
LONDON   NEW YORK   SAN FRANCISCO

A Subsidiary of Harcourt Brace Jovanovich, Publishers

ACADEMIC PRESS INC. (LONDON) LTD.
24–28 Oval Road
London NW1

US edition published by
ACADEMIC PRESS INC.
111 Fifth Avenue,
New York, New York 10003

Library of Congress Catalog Card Number: 64-24672
ISBN: 0-12-013310-5

PRINTED IN GREAT BRITAIN BY
WILLIAM CLOWES & SONS LIMITED
LONDON, COLCHESTER AND BECCLES

Contributors to Volume 10

*W. R. BUCKETT, BPharm, PhD, FPS
Pharmacology Section, Imperial Chemical Industries Ltd, Pharmaceuticals Division, Alderley Park, Cheshire, England

B. DAVIS, BSc, PhD, MIBiol
Pharmacology Department, Glaxo Research Limited, Greenford, Middlesex, England

D. H. METZ, MSc, PhD
National Institute for Medical Research, Mill Hill, London, England

B. F. ROBINSON, MD, FRCP
St. George's Hospital, Hyde Park Corner, London, England

* Present address: Novo A/S, 2880-Bagsvaerd, Copenhagen, Denmark.

Contents

Noninhalational Anaesthetics

B. DAVIS, BSc, PhD, MIBiol

*Pharmacology Department, Glaxo Research Limited,
Greenford, Middlesex, England*

1   Introduction

Attempts to define the sites of action and mechanisms involved in general anaesthesia continue to excite experiment and philosophical discussion (Miller *et al.*, 1965; Halsey and Kent, 1972; Miller *et al.*, 1972b; Anderson and Amaranath, 1973; Eyring *et al.*, 1973; Mullins, 1973; Halsey *et al.*, 1974). With the inhalational anaesthetics there is general recognition that potency can be correlated with lipid solubility, but the search for new anaesthetics still depends upon an empirical approach. This is particularly the case with noninhalational compounds where the possession of lipid solubility is no guarantee of anaesthetic activity. Such compounds must have the right structure as well as being lipid soluble. There is great diversity among the various classes of noninhalational compounds which produce anaesthesia, and their particular properties are the sum of many interacting factors which include lipid solubility, structure, degree of ionization, and the rate and route of metabolism and elimination. These in turn determine potency, speed of onset, duration of action, and degree of cumulation. The qualities which make a compound an acceptable anaesthetic are often not its anaesthetic properties *per se*, but other factors such as its actions on the cardiovascular, respiratory and central nervous systems, and on the body tissues, as well as its stability, and the nature of its degradation products. The noninhalational anaesthetics will be considered predominantly from a pharmacokinetic point of view, but details of clinical activity in animals and man will be included especially with the newer classes of compounds.

Since classical times there have been repeated attempts to produce insensibility during surgery, with alcohol, the opiates, and mandrake, and more recently with chloral hydrate and trichloroethanol. The successful introduction of inhalational anaesthetic agents during the last century eclipsed all these methods. The first real alternative to inhalational anaesthetics occurred with the introduction of the intravenous barbiturates in the 1930s. The intravenous barbiturates were used originally to induce anaesthesia rapidly before transferring to an inhalational agent. More recently, injectable compounds have been developed which alone provide surgical anaesthesia, and some can be used by both the intravenous and intramuscular routes.

The major advantage of an intravenous induction agent is the rapid loss of consciousness after a simple injection. The patient is not subjected to the potentially unpleasant experience of breathing through a face mask while still conscious, which may be resisted by children and animals. The rapidity of onset of anaesthesia is not influenced by breath-holding.

The major disadvantages are that the anaesthetic effect cannot be cut short and a suitable vein must be found. Here again, children and animals may not be cooperative. An intramuscular agent avoids the second problem but speed of induction is sacrificed.

It is easy to list the ideal properties of an intravenous induction agent but difficult to achieve. An ideal anaesthetic would have to have the following properties and be administered in a stable solution containing the human dose in 5 to 10 ml; no pain on injection, local tissue or vascular damage; rapid induction; a wide safety-margin; no cumulation of effect; no respiratory or cardiovascular depression; no laryngospasm or bronchospasm; no twitching or other stimulant activity during induction, sleep or recovery; no dreams or hallucinations; no nausea, vomiting or anorexia; some degree of analgesia; compatibility with all other agents used in anaesthesia. No existing compound satisfies all these criteria.

2 Barbiturates

The sodium salts of amylobarbitone, hexobarbitone and pentobarbitone (Table 1) were the first barbiturates used as intravenous induction agents but were soon succeeded by thiopentone sodium, the thio-analogue of pentobarbitone (Lundy, 1935). Thiopentone has remained the standard induction agent for nearly forty years despite many attempts to displace it. Methohexitone sodium has been the only barbiturate to compete with

TABLE 1

Rapidly acting barbiturates used for induction of anaesthesia by the intravenous route

Name and formula	Structure
Amylobarbitone sodium: sodium 5-ethyl-5-isopentylbarbiturate	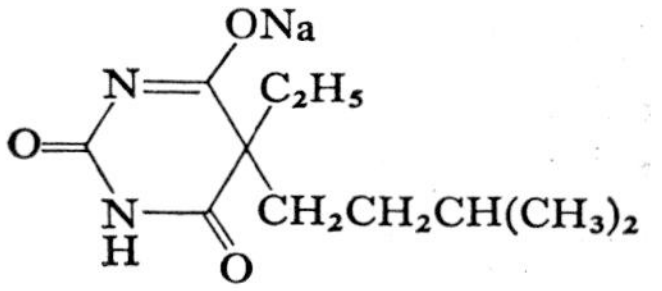
Hexobarbitone sodium: sodium 5-(cyclohex-1-enyl)-1,5-dimethylbarbiturate	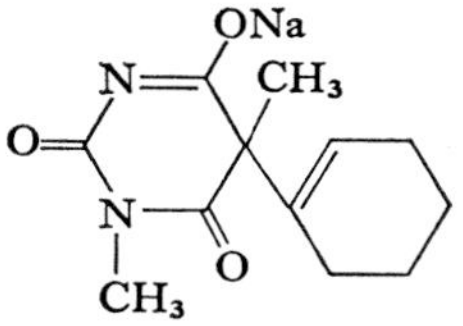
Pentobarbitone sodium: sodium 5-ethyl-5-(1-methylbutyl)-barbiturate	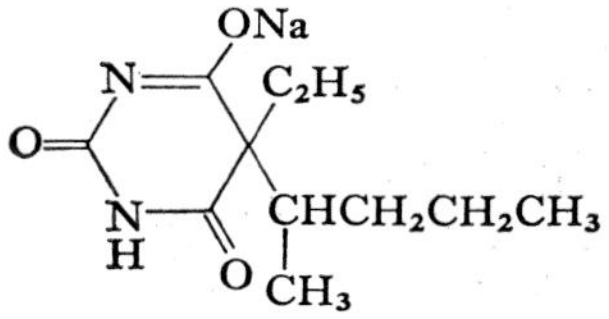
Thiopentone sodium: sodium 5-ethyl-5-(1-methylbutyl)-2-thiobarbiturate	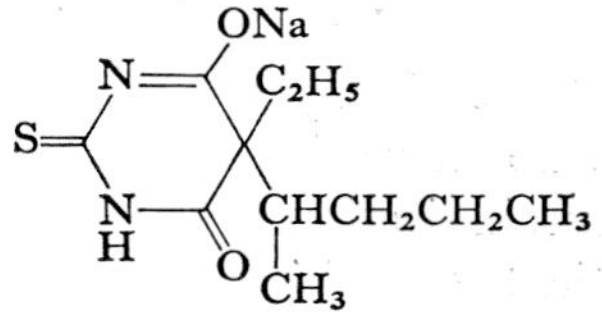
Methohexitone sodium: sodium α-(±)-5-allyl-1-methyl-5-(1-methylpent-2-ynyl)barbiturate	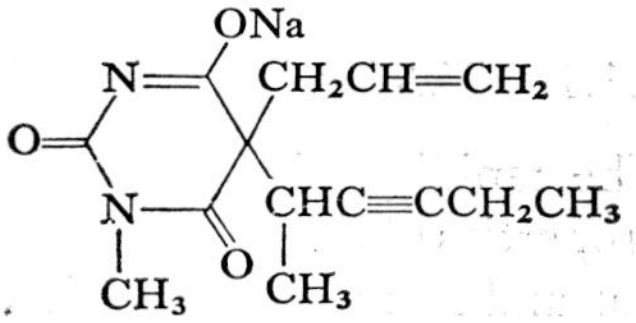

it, and only in recent years have any practical alternatives to the barbiturates appeared.

2.1 THIOPENTONE

The major advantage of thiopentone is the rapidity and smoothness with which it produces loss of consciousness. The time taken is essentially the vein-to-brain circulation time. Spontaneous muscle movement is seen only occasionally after induction and recovery is normally rapid.

Thiopentone has many deficiencies though most are overcome in skilled hands. The aqueous solution of the sodium salt is not very stable and has to be freshly prepared. The solution is very alkaline (about pH 11 for a 5 per cent solution) and this may contribute to the tissue irritation it causes if injected perivenously. The nature of the aqueous solution complicates the effects of accidental intra-arterial injection with thiopentone. It causes severe pain, temporary arterial spasm, and occasionally tissue necrosis in the affected vascular bed (Cohen, 1948a and 1948b). When thiopentone solution is mixed with blood some of the anaesthetic is precipitated from solution (Waters, 1966). In addition, haemolysis and platelet aggregation can occur leading to intravascular thrombosis (Brown et al., 1968). Presumably, by the intravenous route, any precipitated material is soon redissolved by further dilution as its passes into the larger vessels. After accidental intra-arterial injection, the precipitate is swept into vessels of decreasing calibre.

The normal human dose of thiopentone is between 150 and 500 mg but the safety margin is limited. Excessive dosage to overcome the effects of surgical stimulus leads to depression of the respiratory and cardiovascular systems and provides a serious hazard with this anaesthetic (Dundee, 1965a). Safe doses of thiopentone used alone do not provide sufficient analgesia to permit surgery, and some workers consider that with light anaesthesia sensitivity to pain is increased (Clutton Brock, 1960; Dundee, 1960). The laryngospasm that can occur spontaneously or following attempts to intubate the airway may be a result of this increased sensitivity (Paton and Payne, 1968). Post-operative hiccough, nausea and vomiting are no more frequent than after other anaesthetics. The only absolute contraindication to the use of thiopentone, as to other barbiturates, is in patients exhibiting porphyria (Dundee, 1965b).

2.1.1 *Distribution and elimination of thiopentone*

The rapidity of onset, duration of action, safety margin and cumulative properties of thiopentone are determined by the nature of its tissue distribution and eventual elimination from the body, and will therefore be discussed in some detail. They reflect the physicochemical properties of thiopentone, its metabolism, and differences in the blood supply of the various body tissues.

Thiopentone has a pK_a of 7·4 (Bush, 1961) so that about 50 per cent is present in the nonionized form in the blood. The nonionized fraction has high lipid solubility (Bush, 1963) which permits it to pass rapidly into the brain (Price et al., 1957; Mark et al., 1958). Price et al. (1960) showed that in man the brain takes up 10 per cent of an intravenous dose of thiopentone within 1 minute of injection. The brain then loses thiopentone so that after 5 minutes only half the peak concentration remains, and falls to one tenth by 20 minutes. The brevity of action of small doses of thiopentone was originally attributed, on presumptive evidence, to rapid metabolism (Jailer and Goldbaum, 1946), but Brodie et al. (1950) showed that metabolism is slow, and that redistribution into nonnervous tissue, especially fat, is the more probable explanation (Brodie et al., 1952). Redistribution of thiopentone occurs as its equilibrates between the water and fat phases of the tissues. However, the rate of uptake of thiopentone by adipose tissue is too slow to account for the speed with which consciousness is regained (Price et al., 1960), and redistribution initially into other tissues such as muscle has been proposed. It is difficult to obtain direct evidence of the concentration of thiopentone in many tissues at all times during anaesthesia. From the isolated observations available, Price (1960) constructed a mathematical model which predicts the kinetics of thiopentone redistribution. This model provides a satisfactory explanation for all the properties of thiopentone which reflect its disposition and elimination. He suggests that within 1 minute of an intravenous injection of thiopentone, 90 per cent of the dose is distributed into the brain and other organs which receive a rich blood supply. Thereafter the thiopentone is redistributed to other tissues, firstly into lean tissue and then into fat. The rate at which a tissue takes up thiopentone is dependent on the blood supply to the tissue, and the maximum level achieved is dependent on its lipid content. As Price (1960) has suggested, the rate at which the central nervous system loses thiopentone depends predominantly on the rate at which the poorly-perfused tissues gain it. Fat is so slowly perfused that it cannot begin to concentrate thiopentone to an important degree until the central nervous system has already lost over 90 per cent of its peak content. After a single small dose of thiopentone the concentration of thiopentone in the brain falls rapidly below anaesthetic levels as it equilibrates with the blood, and long before equilibrium between the aqueous and lipid tissues is established. Consciousness returns whilst a high proportion of the original dose is still in the body. With repeated doses or slow infusion, more and more tissues approach equilibrium with the thiopentone in the blood during the period of unconsciousness. The capacity of the body tissues to remove thiopentone from the brain is gradually lost (Price, 1960). In such a situation, thiopentone is no longer short-acting, and this explains why repeated doses are increasingly cumulative.

It is generally accepted that eventually thiopentone is eliminated by metabolic degradation in the liver, and that little is excreted unchanged in the urine (Brodie *et al.*, 1950; Mark, 1963). Brodie *et al.* (1950) studied the plasma thiopentone decay curves in human subjects from 1 to 5 hours after intermittent doses of 1 to 4 g. They concluded that the 15 per cent per hour decline in plasma concentration was attributable to metabolic transformation. This assumed negligible urinary excretion, and that equilibrium between the plasma and tissues is established 1 to 2 hours after the original dose. However, the rate of fall of the plasma concentration may not reflect the rate of metabolism accurately. If the tissues were still moving towards equilibrium, the rate of disappearance of thiopentone from the plasma would overestimate the real situation. Alternatively the muscle and fat could provide a reservoir of thiopentone which could, at least in part, replace the metabolized drug, and the rate of disappearance would be underestimated. Despite such considerations, Mark *et al.* (1969) still consider that the plasma decay curves indicate the maximum rate of metabolism of thiopentone. With such an uncertain situation, full balance studies are necessary to discover the true rate of metabolic degradation. One such study in rats (Shideman *et al.*, 1953) indicated that during the first 6 hours, thiopentone was metabolized at a rate of 10 per cent per hour.

How much metabolism influences the duration of anaesthesia with thiopentone is a matter of dispute. Saidman and Eger (1966) have criticized Price (1960) for ignoring it as a factor in the early decline of thiopentone plasma concentrations. They cited studies on the hepatic arterio-venous differences in thiopentone level several hours after dosing, when it was assumed that the tissues were in equilibrium. In their work on dogs, differences of 6·6 and 15·1 per cent were found at 3 and 5 hours respectively, but no information was given about the concentrations measured. Mark *et al.* (1965) showed a 0 to 50 per cent extraction rate by the liver in human patients suffering from various forms of liver disease. Saidman and Eger (1966) concluded from their own results that metabolism plays a significant role in early wakening from anaesthesia. This would appear to be an unsupported conclusion. The ability of the liver to remove an unspecified amount of thiopentone when the concentration is low, gives no indication of its capacity to do so in the early stages of anaesthesia when the concentration is high. There is little evidence that thiopentone is more potent, or has a longer duration of action in patients with liver damage.

Mark *et al.* (1972) referring back to their earlier work (Mark *et al.*, 1965) pointed out that the duration of sleep after thiopentone was similar in all patients regardless of the ability of their livers to remove the drug. There is no direct or circumstantial evidence to suggest how much thiopentone is metabolized in the early stages of anaesthesia. Although liver damage would probably reduce the rate at which thiopentone is metabolized, this is unlikely to influence the duration of anaesthesia after a single dose. It could prolong post-anaesthetic depression and increase the cumulative properties of thiopentone.

Thiopentone is highly protein bound—about 75 per cent at typical plasma concentrations (Brodie *et al.*, 1950). This probably plays a part in the rapid redistribution of thiopentone from the central nervous system and blood into other tissues. Mark *et al.* (1969) suggest that the biodegradation of barbiturates is aided by the high degree of weak protein binding which serves as a transport mechanism to the liver where the barbiturate is easily detached. The slow elimination of the last traces of thiopentone may reflect the increase in protein binding to 90 per cent found when plasma concentrations fall below 5 μg ml^{-1} (Dayton *et al.*, 1967).

It is difficult to predict what effects changes in blood pH will have on the course of thiopentone anaesthesia. Whilst lowering of the pH will increase the proportion of the anaesthetically active nonionized form of thiopentone present in the blood, this is the form which is readily lipid soluble. Brodie *et al.* (1950) showed in the dog that lowering the blood pH several hours after induction of anaesthesia with thiopentone reduced its concentration in the plasma. It is probable that changes in blood pH would influence anaesthesia differently at the early and late stages. Immediately on induction, when the brain and blood concentrations are high, a lowering pH could intensify anaesthesia by increasing the proportion of the active nonionized material available. In the later stages of anaesthesia or during recovery, any lowering of the pH when blood thiopentone concentrations are low, whilst encouraging distribution into fat, would be unlikely to have much influence on the depth of anaesthesia.

2.2 METHOHEXITONE

Methohexitone (Table 1), the only barbiturate to become established as an alternative to thiopentone, is a mixture of the D- and L-α-isomers of sodium 5-allyl-1-methyl-5-(1-methylpent-2-ynyl)barbiturate (25398) (Stoelting, 1957; Gibson *et al.*, 1959). With the original mixture of α- and β-isomers (22451) (Gibson *et al.*, 1955; Gruber *et al.*, 1957) there was a clinically unacceptable occurrence of hiccoughs and muscle tremors. The clinical properties of methohexitone have been described by Taylor and Stoelting (1960). It shares many of the properties of thiopentone but is about three times as potent and has a shorter duration of action. Pain on injection and muscular twitches are the major disadvantages but the incidence of vein damage is possibly less than with thiopentone. Respiratory depression is present at effective anaesthetic doses and may be greater than with equivalent doses of thiopentone. Laryngospasm and coughing are no more frequent than after other barbiturates but the incidence of hiccough is greater. Subsequent work has confirmed the original impressions of methohexitone including the 3:1 potency compared with thiopentone (Clarke et al., 1968) though Barry et al. (1967) have pointed out the problems of comparing potency when duration of action is different. The low incidence of vascular damage with methohexitone may be a consequence of higher potency, as a 1 per cent solution can be used compared with the usual 2·5 per cent solution of thiopentone. It is less cumulative than thiopentone in man (Clarke and Dundee, 1966) and in mice (Child et al., 1971).

The higher potency, shorter duration of action, reduced cumulation and more rapid inactivation of methohexitone probably reflect slight differences in its physicochemical properties compared with thiopentone (Brand et al., 1963). The pK_a of 7·9 and protein binding of 73 per cent for methohexitone compare with 7·4 and 75 per cent for thiopentone. These differences, though slight, mean that more of the active nonionized form of methohexitone is available at blood pH and may explain its higher potency. Further, methohexitone is less lipid soluble than thiopentone and therefore less concentrated in body fat, a site where it would be protected from metabolic transformation. Thus methohexitone has several marginal advantages over thiopentone though these may be outweighed by the greater tendency of methohexitone to produce excitatory phenomena.

2.3   MISCELLANEOUS BARBITURATES

Among the predecessors of thiopentone only pentobarbitone is still in regular use as an intravenous anaesthetic, mainly in animals. It is slightly slower in onset and of longer duration than thiopentone but has an advantage in being formulated as a solution ready for use. Buthalitone, methitural, thialbarbitone and thiamylal (Table 2) have all been claimed to have advantages over thiopentone but none has proved sufficiently different to displace it (Dundee, 1963, 1971).

Thiohexital (Table 2), the desmethyl thio-analogue of methohexitone is the most recent barbiturate to be examined clinically (Mark et al., 1968). It is considered the most rapidly metabolized barbiturate (25 per cent per hour in man) and has a shorter duration of action than methohexitone. Side effects in man include twitching, tremors and hiccough, and it has been

TABLE 2

Miscellaneous rapidly acting barbiturates used for induction of anaesthesia by the intravenous route

Name and formula	Structure
Buthalitone sodium: sodium 5-allyl-5-isobutyl-2-thiobarbiturate	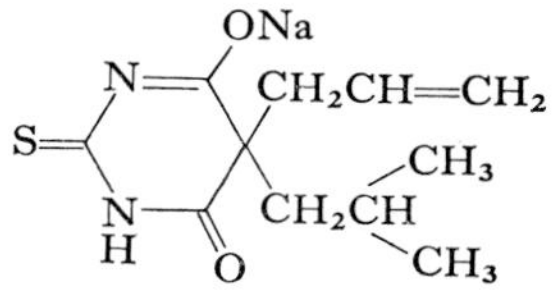 ONa; N; S; N–H; O; $CH_2CH{=}CH_2$; $CH_2CH\,{<}^{CH_3}_{CH_3}$
Methitural sodium: sodium 5-(1-methylbutyl)-5-(2-(methylthio)ethyl)-2-thiobarbiturate	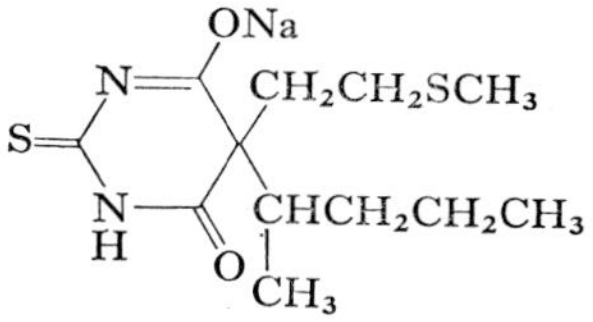 ONa; N; S; N–H; O; $CH_2CH_2SCH_3$; $CHCH_2CH_2CH_3$ with CH_3
Thialbarbitone sodium: sodium 5-allyl-5-(cyclohex-2-enyl)-2-thiobarbiturate	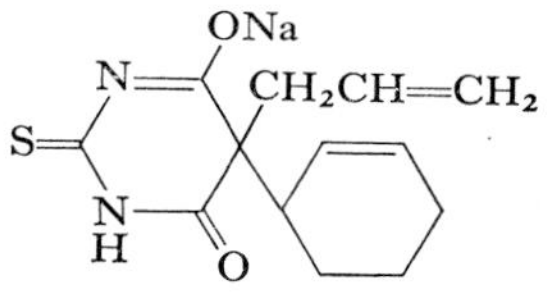 ONa; N; S; N–H; O; $CH_2CH{=}CH_2$; cyclohexenyl ring
Thiamylal sodium: sodium 5-allyl-5-(1-methylbutyl)-2-thiobarbiturate	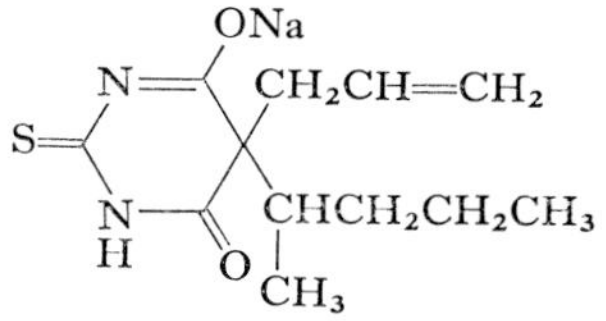 ONa; N; S; N–H; O; $CH_2CH{=}CH_2$; $CHCH_2CH_2CH_3$ with CH_3
Thiohexital sodium: sodium 5-allyl-5-(1-methylpent-2-ynyl)-2-thiobarbiturate	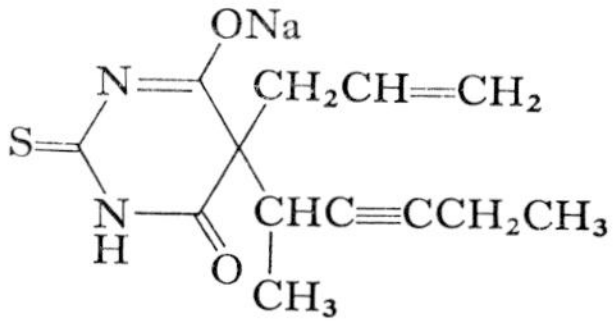 ONa; N; S; N–H; O; $CH_2CH{=}CH_2$; $CHC{\equiv}CCH_2CH_3$ with CH_3

suggested that, as was found during the development of methohexitone, one of its stereo isomers might produce less of these undesirable effects.

2.4 CONCLUSIONS ON BARBITURATES

The relative failure to improve upon thiopentone, despite the testing of many thousands of barbiturates, testifies to the difficulty in finding the perfect anaesthetic in this class of compounds. The necessity to use strongly alkaline solutions is an important disadvantage of the barbiturates. However their major flaw—cumulation of action with repeated doses—arises because their duration of action is controlled by redistribution rather than metabolism. Unless a new barbiturate is developed which is metabolized at a very much faster rate than existing compounds, there will be no real advance in this class of intravenous anaesthetics.

3 Gamma-hydroxybutyric acid

Gamma-hydroxybutyric acid (sodium 4-hydroxybutyrate) (**1**), commonly known as Gamma OH, was introduced into anaesthesia by Laborit *et al.* (1960). They considered it might act by entering into the metabolic pathway of the putative central nervous system inhibitor gamma-aminobutyric acid (GABA) (**2**). Gamma OH produced sleep when given by the oral and by the

$$HOCH_2CH_2CH_2COONa \qquad\qquad H_2NCH_2CH_2CH_2COOH$$

$$(1) \qquad\qquad\qquad\qquad\qquad (2)$$

intravenous routes but it has not become widely accepted as an anaesthetic except in France (Vickers, 1969). The dose of Gamma OH is high (4 to 6 g), the onset of unconsciousness is slow (10 to 20 minutes even after intravenous injection), and it does not produce true surgical anaesthesia when used alone. It is best regarded as a basal anaesthetic and clearly has none of the essential properties of an induction agent.

4 Phenylcyclohexylamine derivatives

The quality of anaesthesia produced by the phenylcyclohexylamine derivatives differs from that of all other anaesthetics. They produce a state resembling catalepsy rather than sedation or hypnosis particularly in lower doses. It has been suggested that the reactivity of the central nervous system to sensory stimuli is altered but not truly blocked. Although sensory input may reach cortical areas, they fail to be perceived in some of the association areas which are depressed. The state produced by the phenylcyclohexylamine anaesthetics therefore has been called "dissociative anaesthesia" (Corssen and Domino, 1966). This difference in action makes comparison with conventional anaesthetics difficult as some of the usual criteria for assessing depth of anaesthesia are not present.

4.1 PHENCYCLIDINE

Phencyclidine, 1-(1-phenylcyclohexyl)piperidine hydrochloride (**3**), was the first compound of this class to be evaluated in animals and man. In most species, phencyclidine produces a combination of stimulation and depression, stimulation being most prominent with lower doses in mice and rats. A gradation of effect from catalepsy towards a state of general anaesthesia is seen in cats, dogs and monkeys, though convulsions are seen with

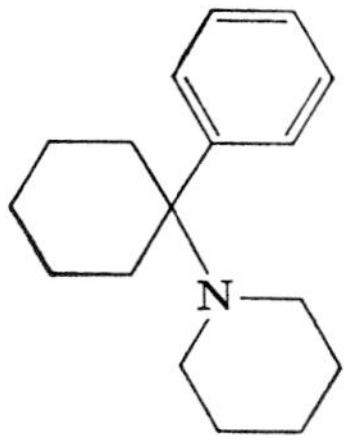

HCl

(3)

higher doses in these species. (Chen *et al.*, 1959). Blood pressure is usually slightly raised, respiration is depressed only at the higher doses, and there is some local anaesthetic effect. Phencyclidine is active by the intravenous and the intramuscular routes. It was used particularly in the management of monkeys (Chen and Weston, 1960) and, despite its long duration of action, it was used in a wide range of zoo animals (Kroll, 1962).

In man, phencyclidine proved unsatisfactory because of marked psychotomimetic actions and often prolonged post-anaesthetic confusion (Johnstone *et al.*, 1959).

4.2 KETAMINE

Ketamine (2-(*o*-chlorophenyl)-2-methylaminocyclohexanone hydrochloride) (4) succeeded phencyclidine. Ketamine is less potent, is of shorter

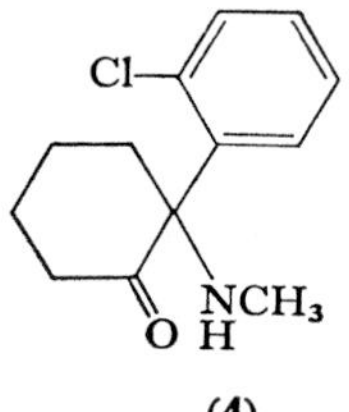

Cl

HCl

NCH₃

O H

(4)

duration, and less stimulant than phencyclidine yet possesses the same type of anaesthetic action. McCarthy *et al.* (1965) compared the properties of phencyclidine and ketamine with those of two barbiturates, pentobarbitone and thiamylal, in laboratory animals. They found that with ketamine the central nervous system was predominantly depressed. The animals passed through a state of catalepsy into general anaesthesia with increasing doses though the effects were different from those of conventional anaesthetics. Induction was rapid though slightly slower than with the barbiturates. Cats and dogs showed muscular rigidity, salivation and urination. Their eyes were usually open, dilated, and showed nystagmus. Pharyngeal reflexes were not depressed. Monkeys were the species in which ketamine produced the best quality of anaesthesia. In unanaesthetized dogs, ketamine produced dose-related rises in blood pressure, and little respiratory depression except at the highest dose levels. Cardiovascular collapse and respiratory depression were marked when ketamine was injected into animals already anaesthetized with pentobarbitone or chloralose. This is an effect similar to that reported with steroid anaesthetics (Lerman and Paton, 1960; Child et al., 1972a).

The first use of ketamine in man was described by Corssen and Domino (1966). As well as recognizing qualitative differences in the responses to ketamine, they found induction slightly slower than with conventional rapidly acting anaesthetics. Adequate anaesthesia was obtained in 1 to $1\frac{1}{2}$ minutes after the start of an intravenous dose of 1 to 2 mg kg^{-1} and lasted for 5 to 8 minutes. Arterial pressure rose, particularly if the injection rate was rapid and this also increased the slight initial respiratory depression. The rise in blood pressure varied from "trivial" in some patients to "alarming" in others. The protective pharyngeal, laryngeal, eyelid and corneal reflexes, as well as pronounced muscle tone, were present throughout anaesthesia but analgesia was presumed to be quite adequate. Recovery was moderately rapid, and was accompanied in a significant number of patients by vivid dreams or hallucinations some of which were unpleasant. By the intramuscular route, an acceptable degree of anaesthesia and analgesia was obtained with doses of 4 to 5 mg kg^{-1} in about 5 to 8 minutes and lasted for 20 to 30 minutes.

All subsequent studies in man have confirmed these initial findings. Virtue et al. (1967) remarked on the excellent analgesic action of ketamine, and showed that despite rises in blood pressure the myocardium was not sensitized to the effects of adrenaline. Szappanyos et al. (1969) found ketamine particularly useful for children in whom they found a much lower incidence of psychic side effects than in adults. They also found little cumulation with ketamine as it was possible to give repeated doses of half the initial dose without prolongation of action. The latter finding is not in agreement with that of Corssen et al. (1968) who found recovery prolonged after multiple supplementary doses. Dundee et al. (1970) found that half the patients induced with 2 mg kg^{-1} of ketamine intravenously as the sole agent required further doses but this was not necessary after 3 mg kg^{-1}.

One third of all adult patients were disturbed by their experiences during recovery, but no post-operative delirium or hallucinations were recorded in children. The detailed and clear description of the effects of ketamine in man by Morgan et al. (1971) serves to summarize its properties. They administered 2 to 2·2 mg kg⁻¹ intravenously as a 1 per cent solution over 45 to 60 seconds. Some patients received up to a maximum of 9 repeated doses without signs of cumulation. Induction was smooth and most patients appeared asleep 30 to 40 seconds after the end of the injection. The eyes then reopened and remained so, often accompanied at first by nystagmus. The eyes always closed before a further dose of ketamine was required. Children usually received 10 to 20 mg kg⁻¹ of ketamine as a 5 per cent solution by the intramuscular route. Here surgery was started after 5 minutes and recovery times were longer than after intravenous doses. The generalized increase in muscle tone and purposeless movements during operation were rarely troublesome. Heart rate and blood pressure were stimulated, reaching a maximum 3 to 4 minutes after the first intravenous injection but subsequent doses had little effect. Most patients appeared to go into natural sleep for periods of up to 4 hours after return to the ward, and none had any recollection of the surgical procedure. Emergence reactions in adults included vivid dreams and vocalization during recovery. Ten per cent of patients had such frightening dreams that they would not wish to have the same anaesthetic again. Corssen et al. (1968) had found the incidence of emergence reactions less if the patients were not stimulated during recovery but Morgan et al. (1971) questioned the propriety of dispensing with the customary surveillance procedures.

Psychic phenomena are not definable in animals but catatonia and trance-like states, as well as undesirable side effects such as urination and excessive salivation are readily recognized after ketamine in most species (Child et al., 1972a; Reid and Frank, 1972; Glen, 1973). In pigs, excitement has led to death following hyperpyrexia in strains susceptible to the "porcine stress" syndrome (Thurmon et al., 1972).

The major advantages of ketamine are its efficacy by both the intravenous and intramuscular routes, its good analgesia, and the maintenance of laryngeal and pharyngeal reflexes, though Taylor et al. (1972) and Carson et al. (1973) have demonstrated that ketamine produces some incompetence of these reflexes. The stimulant actions on the cardiovascular system are generally accepted as beneficial except where there is an obvious contra-indication as in hypertension (Tweed et al., 1972). The rise in blood pressure probably results from sympathetic stimulation as the plasma catecholamine levels rise by as much as 50 per cent 2 minutes after intravenous administration of ketamine (Takki et al., 1972). There is a marked rise in intracranial pressure and cerebrospinal fluid pressure (Gibbs,

1972; List *et al.*, 1972; Wyte *et al.*, 1972) but this may be terminated with a dose of thiopentone (Shapiro *et al.*, 1972).

Despite some conflict of evidence already mentioned, on balance ketamine shows little tendency to cumulation though recovery can be prolonged. Ketamine is rapidly absorbed and distributed throughout the body after both parenteral and oral administration. Experiments in rats (Chang *et al.*, 1965) show the highest concentrations of ketamine to be in body fat. These levels are 10 times those in plasma, with liver, lung, spleen, kidney, brain, heart and skeletal muscle occupying intermediate positions in descending order. Only small amounts of unchanged ketamine are found in the urine. Two metabolic products, the demethylated primary amine (metabolite I) (5), and the primary amine oxidized to the cyclohexene derivative (metabolite II) have been isolated from monkey urine. Metabolite II is the major product in the urine of man, monkeys and dogs, whilst metabolite I (5) and an unidentified compound predominate in rat urine. Recent work in rats using gas–liquid chromatography techniques (Cohen *et al.*, 1973) shows that metabolite I (5) accumulates in the brain in higher concentrations than in the plasma 10 minutes after injection. It is therefore suggested that metabolite I (5) could be responsible for the later central nervous system effects of ketamine. Tritium-labelled ketamine administered to man intravenously at a dose of 1 mg kg^{-1} yields peak plasma tritium levels 3 to 5 minutes after the dose (Chang *et al.*, 1970). A second peak plasma level occurs 1 to 2 hours later. This result appears to reflect rapid uptake by the tissues followed by a slow return of the metabolites. Ninety-one per cent of the administered tritium was recovered from the urine and 3 per cent from the faeces in the 5 days after dosing. The biological half-life of ketamine in the plasma was calculated as 4 hours by these authors, but subsequently Chang and Glazko (1972) using a GLC technique found a quite different half-life of 17 minutes. Other recent studies in man show the major metabolite in the plasma 1 hour after dosing to be the primary amine hydroxylated at the 3-position of the cyclohexanone ring (metabolite III). The urine, as well as containing metabolites I and II, also contains metabolite IV which is another polar compound similar to metabolite III but hydroxylated at the 4-position (Dill *et al.*, 1971).

(5)

The major disadvantage of ketamine is the relatively high incidence of unpleasant dreams and psychic effects seen post-operatively. These have been likened in some cases to the effects of marihuana and LSD (Collier, 1972). All authors agree that these effects are most unacceptable in young and middle-aged adults, and are quite uncommon in children and the elderly. There is some evidence that the incidence of psychic phenomena is low in non-European populations (Walker, 1972).

It must be concluded that ketamine, whilst providing a new dimension in anaesthesia, produces effects which prevent it from being fully acceptable.

5 Eugenol derivatives

Derivatives of eugenol (4-allyl-2-methoxyphenol) (6) were the first non-barbiturates to produce rapid induction of anaesthesia of short duration by the intravenous route. Though possessing several of the desirable properties of the barbiturates, the eugenols have the advantage of being noncumulative. The discovery of their anaesthetic properties resulted from a general pharmacodynamic evaluation of a series of hydrolysable esters of phenoxyacetic acid amides derived from eugenol (Hiltmann et al., 1965).

Two seemingly incompatible physicochemical properties are necessary for a rapidly acting intravenous anaesthetic, namely high lipid solubility and water solubility. With the barbiturates this is achieved by using aqueous solutions of the sodium salts at a high pH. Presumably the eugenol derivatives which are mostly oils do not form suitable water-soluble salts, and other methods of solubilization using organic solvents or solubilizing agents are needed.

5.1 G29.505

The first eugenol derivative to be widely tested as an anaesthetic G29.505 (2-methoxy-4-allylphenoxyacetic acid N,N-diethylamide) (7) was originally formulated in propylene glycol and sodium benzoate. It rapidly induced anaesthesia of short duration by the intravenous route in a variety of species (Thuillier and Domenjoz, 1957). Subsequently it was tested in animals and man as an emulsion prepared with lecithin. With such a formulation, onset of anaesthesia in animals was accompanied by bradycardia, a fall in blood pressure, hyperventilation followed by apnoea, and in some cases haemorrhagic pulmonary oedema (Payne and Wright, 1962). The pulmonary oedema was attributed to the solvent though the solvent alone produced no such effect. It would seem more probable that the physical

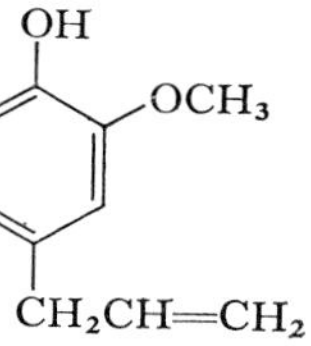

OH
OCH₃
CH₂CH=CH₂
(6)

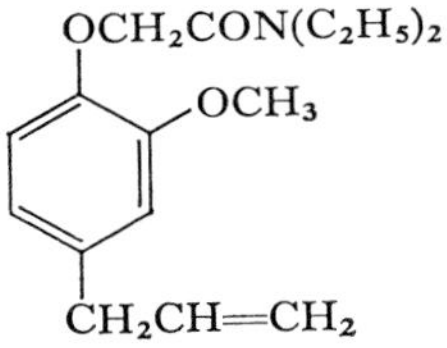

OCH₂CON(C₂H₅)₂
OCH₃
CH₂CH=CH₂
(7)

form of the emulsion was responsible, in the light of results by Corssen (1964). He demonstrated multiple fat droplets in biopsy specimens of the lungs of dogs taken at the peak of the hyperventilatory phase. Repeated doses had less and less hyperventilatory effect—a tachyphylactic phenomenon commonly observed when particulate matter is injected intravenously. In man, this emulsified formulation of G29.505, though producing a transient respiratory stimulant effect followed by brief apnoea, had little effect on the heart rate or blood pressure (Swerdlow, 1961, 1962; Wright and Payne, 1962).

G29.505, though useful for its rapidity of onset and short duration of anaesthesia, proved unacceptable because of its irritant effects on the vascular system in a high proportion of patients (Swerdlow, 1962; Riding *et al.*, 1963; Frey, 1971).

5.2   PROPINAL

A closely related eugenol derivative propinal (2-methoxy-4-propyl phenoxyacetic acid *N*,*N*-diethylamide) (**8**) had similar properties to G29.505. Though it was claimed to be free of vascular irritant effects, no further publications on work with this compound have been traced since it was first tested by Nishimura (1962).

5.3   PROPANIDID

Propanidid (propyl 4-diethyl-carbamoylmethoxy-3-methoxyphenyl acetate) (**9**) was the first eugenol derivative to be used on a wide scale in anaesthesia. Though propandid is an oil, a 5 per cent solution miscible with water can be achieved by dissolving it in a 20 per cent solution of the nonionic surface-active agent Cremophor EL ® (polyoxyethylated castor oil). More recently Micellophor, a 16 per cent solution of the hydrophobic fraction of Cremophor EL, has been used as the solvent, as it gives a less viscous solution. These formulations of propanidid, whilst possessing anaesthetic properties similar to G29.505, produce much less vascular irritation.

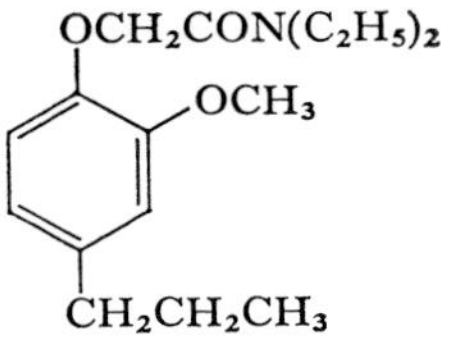

OCH$_2$CON(C$_2$H$_5$)$_2$

OCH$_3$

CH$_2$CH$_2$CH$_3$

(8)

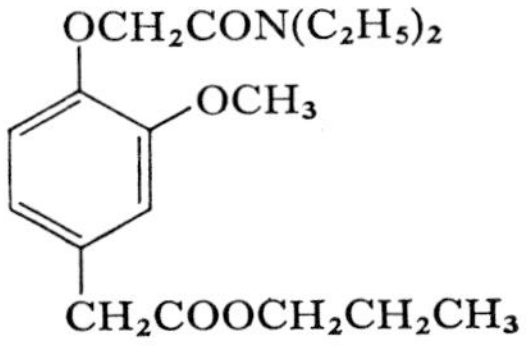

OCH$_2$CON(C$_2$H$_5$)$_2$

OCH$_3$

CH$_2$COOCH$_2$CH$_2$CH$_3$

(9)

5.3.1   Animal pharmacology of propanidid

The pharmacological properties of propanidid have been described by Wirth and Hoffmeister (1965). Anaesthesia is induced in the vein-to-brain circulation time by the intravenous route in mice, rats, rabbits, dogs and monkeys. The potency of propanidid is similar to that of thiopentone. The duration of anaesthesia is short and animals return to normal rapidly. The blood pressure falls during the first few minutes mainly as a result of peripheral vasodilatation but usually returns to normal within 3 to 10 minutes. The early stages of anaesthesia are accompanied by hyperventilation which is followed in the higher doses by a period of apnoea. There is no evidence of analgesia or anti-analgesia, though propanidid has a definite local anaesthetic action when injected into the tissues. Propanidid is moderately well tolerated locally and intravenously in all species. However, in the dog propanidid produces an anaphylactoid response with the release of histamine and other vaso-active substances. This response is manifested after a delay of 2 to 3 minutes. The skin becomes pink and blotchy with some oedema and evidence of pruritus. The dog may retch, vomit or defaecate, and there is a fall in blood pressure. The anaphylactoid response is attributable to the solubilizing agent Cremophor EL. It is typical of the response of this species and of other members of the genus Canis to a wide variety of polymeric compounds (Krantz et al., 1948; Krantz et al., 1949). Some of the cardiovascular studies on propanidid are difficult to interpret where they have been carried out in dogs. Thus Conway et al. (1968) carried out a careful comparison of the haemodynamic effects of thiopentone, methohexitone and propanidid in this species, giving results irrelevant to man. The responses of man and dogs to barbiturates are similar, whereas their responses to propanidid differ. Further, the reaction of the dog to a first dose of propanidid is different in nature and degree from its reaction to subsequent doses. Only after an interval of about 24 hours does the dog respond to a further dose in a way similar to its initial reaction. The experiments of Langrehr (1965) are open to a similar criticism, and here, possible interactions with other anaesthetics are an added complication.

Propanidid has not been used on a wide scale for anaesthesia in animals because of its brevity of action. Child *et al.* (1972a) in a comparative study of intravenous anaesthetics in cats were unable to produce surgical anaesthesia with propanidid.

5.3.2 *Clinical pharmacology of propanidid*

An early clinical comparison of propanidid with G29.505, methohexitone and thiopentone in man soon established its main properties (Dundee and Clarke, 1964). The rather viscous solution induced anaesthesia rapidly and smoothly followed by some hyperventilation and a low incidence of excitatory phenomena. The induction dose of 4·1 mg kg^{-1} for propanidid was similar to that for thiopentone. The duration of anaesthesia with propanidid was shorter with a more rapid return to clear headedness, and there was no cumulation of effect with repeated doses. Post-operative nausea and vomiting were more common than with barbiturates during the first hour of recovery but not significantly different during the next 5 hours. No particular hypotensive action was noted, and vascular irritation was much less than after G29.505. Howells *et al.* (1964), using doses of 5 and 10 mg kg^{-1} considered the lower dose of propanidid insufficient in some patients. Their general conclusions were in agreement with those of Dundee and Clarke (1964) and provided further points of detail. The hyperventilatory phase which lasted for up to 30 seconds, was usually followed by a period of apnoea of up to 1 minute after the 10 mg kg^{-1} dose. These authors found a fall in blood pressure of about 30 per cent and a tachycardia accompanying or sometimes preceding the hyperventilatory phase. There was no consistent evidence of an analgesic or anti-analgesic action, but there was a definite local-anaesthetic action if a small volume of propanidid was injected perivenously. No nausea or vomiting was seen in patients given propanidid as the sole anaesthetic. These authors also confirmed an observation of Dundee that propanidid potentiated the neuromuscular blocking action of suxamethonium. More patients are apnoeic for longer periods after suxamethonium if anaesthetized with propanidid than those anaesthetized with methohexitone or thiopentone. However, there is a large overlap in the response to suxamethonium regardless of the anaesthetic (Clark *et al.*, 1967). The exact mechanisms are uncertain and could involve interference with the metabolism of suxamethonium or with its neuromuscular blocking properties. It is possible that propanidid competes with cholinesterases in the blood but the evidence for this is equivocal (Doenicke *et al.*, 1968). In patients anaesthetized with thiopentone, nitrous oxide and halothane, the intensity of suxamethonium-induced neuromuscular block is slightly potentiated by propanidid. The time to maximum block and the duration of block are increased significantly and out of proportion to the increase in intensity. The block after decamethonium is neither potentiated nor prolonged, and it is suggested that the hydrolysis rate of suxamethonium is reduced (Torda *et al.*, 1972). Monks and Norman (1972) have also found a prolongation of suxamethonium neuromuscular blockade after propanidid.

There is general agreement that in man a 4 mg kg^{-1} dose of propanidid produces a low incidence of hypotension similar to that with the same dose of thiopentone or an equivalent dose of methohexitone. Above 8 mg kg^{-1} of propanidid the incidence and severity of hypotension increase beyond clinically acceptable levels (Clarke, 1969). Henschel and Buhr (1965) showed that with an intravenous dose of 500 mg of propanidid in man, there is an immediate fall in systolic blood pressure of up to 40 mmHg accompanied by an increase in heart rate, a fall in stroke volume, and a reduction in peripheral resistance. There is a return to normal by the end of anaesthesia in 5 to 6 minutes. Johnstone and Barron (1968), using radio-telemetric techniques in man, suggested that the hypotension is cardiac in origin and unrelated to peripheral vasodilatation. They found definite electrocardiographic evidence of an initial quinidine-like cardiac depression but this was rapidly overcome by reflex tachycardia associated with the hypotension. When comparing the cardiovascular effects of propanidid (7 mg kg^{-1}) and methohexitone (2 mg kg^{-1}) intravenously in patients anaesthetized with nitrous oxide, Beer and Soga (1971) found a reduction of the mean arterial pressure of 30 per cent after propanidid, resulting predominantly from myocardial depression and to a lesser extent from a decrease in peripheral resistance. The initial increase in heart rate was insufficient to compensate for the reduced stroke volume. With methohexitone, arterial pressure remained within normal limits and though there was a persistent reduction in vascular resistance, depression of cardiac contractility was only transient. A recent comparison of propanidid and methohexitone in healthy volunteers is in substantial agreement (Bernhoff *et al.*, 1972).

The hyperventilatory action of propanidid is associated with the active constituent and not the solubilizing agent, and is effected via a stimulation of the carotid sinus (Gordh, 1971). There is no possibility that part of the action results from the formation of micro-emboli in the lungs as occurred with the G29.505 emulsion.

Propanidid is much less likely to produce vascular irritant effects than G29.505 but it causes slightly more venous complications than thiopentone and methohexitone (Hewitt *et al.*, 1966). Hoffmeister *et al.* (1965), and Weis and Ruckes (1965) compared propanidid with thiopentone using various intra-arterial injection methods in animals. They concluded that propanidid was slightly better tolerated than thiopentone and that the

2·5 per cent of solutions of both anaesthetics caused less damage than the 5 per cent solutions. A more extensive study in animals and man of the short- and long-term effects of intra-arterial injection of propanidid into limbs described the circulatory and histo-pathological changes. Under normal conditions in man there was no permanent vascular damage using the doses of propanidid required for short operations (Liebegott, 1965).

5.3.3   Potency and fate of propanidid

Clarke *et al.* (1968) have compared the induction doses of propanidid, methohexitone and thiopentone. They first reviewed the methods for estimating potency, and pointed out that equipotent induction doses should not be confused with doses producing anaesthesia of equal duration. To overcome variations in vein-to-brain circulation time, the induction agents were injected during the period of reactive hyperaemia following vascular occlusion. They found the doses where 90 per cent of patients were unable to continue counting 11 seconds after the end of injection. Propanidid was very slightly less potent than thiopentone, and methohexitone was three times as potent, giving minimum anaesthetic induction doses of 3·35 mg kg^{-1} for propanidid, 3·0 mg kg^{-1} for thiopentone and 0·95 mg kg^{-1} for methohexitone. The relationship between dosage and duration of sleep with propanidid has been studied by Clarke (1968) over the range 0·8 to 15·2 mg kg^{-1} in female patients premedicated with 0·65 mg of atropine. There was an almost linear relationship though the duration of sleep did not continue to increase in proportion to the dose. The longest period of sleep after a single dose was about 6 minutes and surgical anaesthesia was shorter. An earlier comparative study which assessed the doses producing unresponsiveness in 50 per cent of patients for 1, 3 and 4 minutes gave figures of 3·5, 6·8 and 9·9 mg kg^{-1} for propanidid, and 0·64, 1·31 and 1·65 mg kg^{-1} for methohexitone (Howells *et al.*, 1967).

These and similar clinical observations show that propanidid is truly short-acting. The lack of cumulation with repeated doses is confirmed by the experiments of Clarke and Dundee (1966). Anaesthesia was maintained in patients for at least 1 hour by an induction dose of either propanidid, thiopentone or methohexitone followed by intermittent doses of the same anaesthetics as required. There was a marked falling off of the requirements for the barbiturates but little decline with propanidid.

It is clear that the brevity of action of propanidid is governed by its rapid metabolism and not primarily by redistribution as occurs with the barbiturates. In man, plasma levels of propanidid are undetectable 25 minutes after an intravenous dose of 7 mg kg^{-1} (Doenicke *et al.*, 1968). In rats, the biological half-life of ^{14}C-labelled propanidid is 20 minutes and

90 per cent of the dose is found in the urine in the form of metabolites within 2 hours (Duhm *et al.*, 1965). Most of the propanidid is excreted as the inactive 3-methoxy-4-*N*,*N*-diethylcarbamidomethoxyphenylacetic acid (10). The ester bond in propanidid is hydrolysed by esterases in the plasma of man and some animals, as well as in the liver of all species (Pütter,

$$OCH_2CON(C_2H_5)_2$$

$$OCH_3$$

$$CH_2COOH$$

(10)

1965). It is possible that the cholinesterases are involved, and though *in vitro* and *in vivo* experiments using cholinesterase inhibitors have not supported this view (Wirth and Hoffmeister, 1965; Doenicke *et al.*, 1965), Doenicke *et al.* (1968) have pointed out that inappropriate species, or insufficiently inhibitory doses of anti-cholinesterase were used.

Propanidid is protein-bound to the extent of 70·1 per cent (Kurz, 1966). In patients with a low plasma protein concentration, propanidid is more potent and anaesthesia is of longer duration than in normal patients (Doenicke *et al.*, 1968).

5.3.4 *Hypersensitivity reactions to propanidid*

There have been an increasing number of reports of hypersensitivity reactions to propanidid in recent years. Kruger (1970) referred to 14 previous cases and described 2 more, whilst Jarvis (1972), Rozenkranz (1972) and Turner *et al.* (1972) each reported one case. Reactions were reported in some cases following a first administration but in others they occurred only after a second or subsequent dose. Lorenz *et al.* (1972) have carried out a careful study of this phenomenon. Intravenous doses of propanidid or thiopentone in the clinical range in normal subjects cause a rise in the plasma histamine level to about 350 per cent of normal in 5 minutes which returns to normal by 30 minutes. The solvents used for propanidid (Cremophor EL or Micellophor) cause a rise of only 20 per cent, and the solvent for thiopentone (0·9 per cent sodium chloride) is without effect. In patients showing an anaphylactoid reaction to propanidid the rises in plasma histamine level are much greater than in normal subjects. Furthermore, these patients only show the small rise in plasma histamine after Cremophor EL or Micellophor, so these solvents cannot be the direct cause of any reaction. The amount of histamine released by propanidid or thiopentone in normal subjects is insufficient to cause the tachycardia and hypotension normally seen after these drugs, and the time course of its release is inappropriate. It is probable that in most patients showing a hypersensitivity reaction to propanidid there is massive histamine release. Other vaso-active substances may be released but they have not been studied. Many of the effects of propanidid in sensitive patients may be mitigated by the use of corticosteroids and plasma expanders. Existing antihistamine drugs are only partially effective but it is possible that the recently described inhibitor of histamine H2 receptors, burimamide (Black *et al.*, 1972), may add to their effectiveness. The true incidence and significance of reactions to propanidid have not been fully assessed, but as Frey (1971) pointed out, propanidid has already been used in over 20 million anaesthetic procedures throughout the world.

5.3.5 *Conclusions on propanidid*

There can be no doubt that propanidid provided the first rapidly acting anaesthetic of short duration as an alternative to the barbiturates. In addition it is free of any tendency to cumulate, and unlike the barbiturates, it is not contraindicated in porphyria (Dean, 1969). It is clear that propanidid is not the ideal induction agent because of several minor deficiencies in its properties, and the necessity to use a solubilizing agent to achieve an injectable solution. However, it has demonstrated that most of the desirable properties of an induction agent are not confined to the barbiturates and can be sought elsewhere.

6 Steroid anaesthetics

6.1 NOMENCLATURE

To avoid ambiguity in naming the steroids, the conventional numbering of the carbon atoms and lettering of the rings are used (Fig. 1). The spatial conformation of the molecules is indicated by the configuration at key positions, e.g. at carbon 5. The symbol α indicates substituents projecting below the plane of the molecule and is drawn as a dotted line, and β indicates substituents projecting above the plane of the molecule and is drawn as a solid line. Thus 3α-hydroxy-5α-pregnane-11,20-dione and 3α-hydroxy-5β-pregnane-11,20-dione are drawn conventionally as in Fig. 2. The three-dimensional character of molecules can be represented diagrammatically as in Fig. 3. Terms such as allo- for the 5α-configuration (with the ring A/B junction *trans*), or normal for the 5β-configuration (with the ring A/B

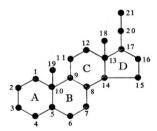

FIG. 1. The numbering of the carbon atoms, and lettering of the rings of steroid molecules.

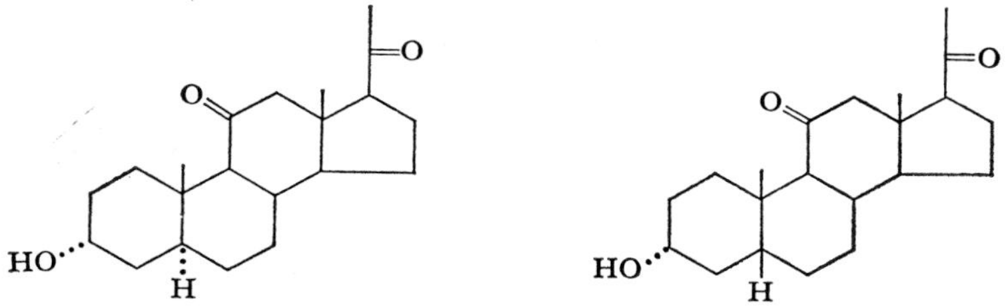

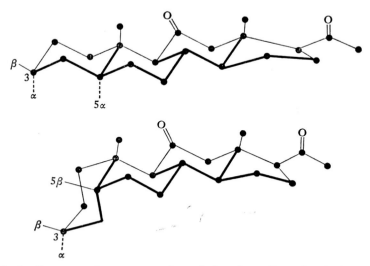

FIG. 2. The conventional representation of 3α-hydroxy-5α-pregnane-11,20-dione and 3α-hydroxy-5β-pregnane-11,20-dione.

FIG. 3. A diagrammatic representation of the three-dimensional character of steroid molecules with the 5α- or 5β-configuration. Substituents at 3-, and most of the hydrogen atoms are omitted for clarity.

junction *cis*) will not be used. Trivial names are used for well-known compounds such as progesterone and testosterone.

6.2   DISCOVERY OF STEROID ANAESTHESIA

The discovery of the anaesthetic activity of certain steroids was not the result of a deliberate search for this property. Selye (1941a) had noticed how difficult it was to produce acute overdosage phenomena with highly potent steroid hormones. He speculated that this might be the result of slow absorption of these water-insoluble compounds after subcutaneous injection. To circumvent this he dissolved them in peanut oil and injected them intraperitoneally into male and female rats. Unexpectedly the female rats became deeply anaesthetized 15 minutes after injection of progesterone (**11**) or desoxycorticosterone acetate (**12**), and 1 hour after testosterone (**13**). Male rats were much less affected, and oestradiol (**14**) and cholesterol

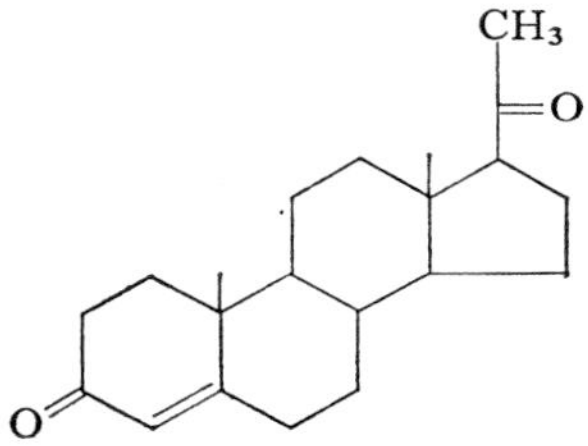

(11)

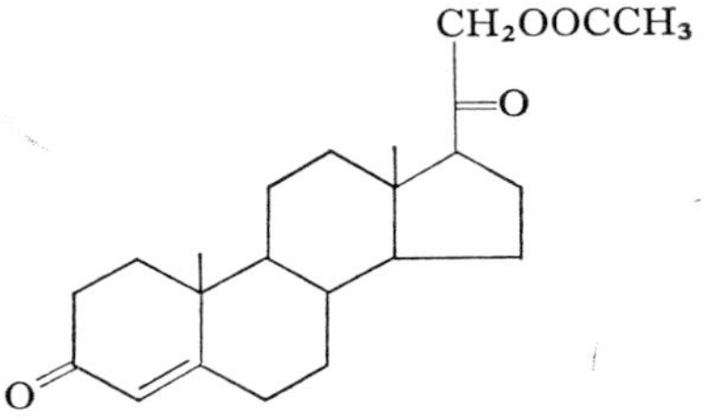

(12)

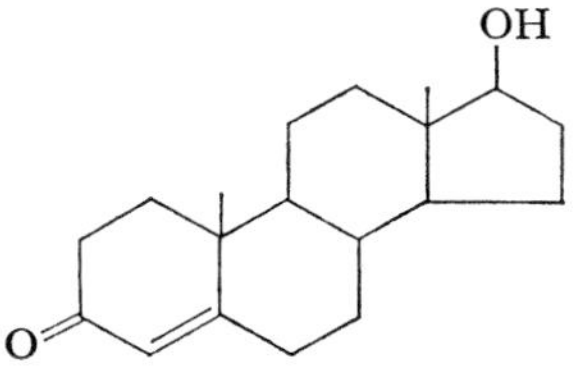

(13)

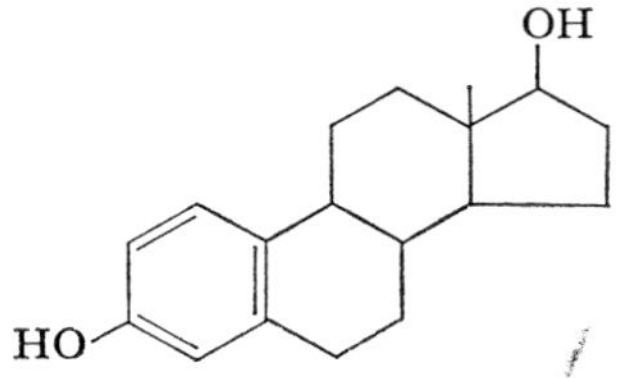

(14)

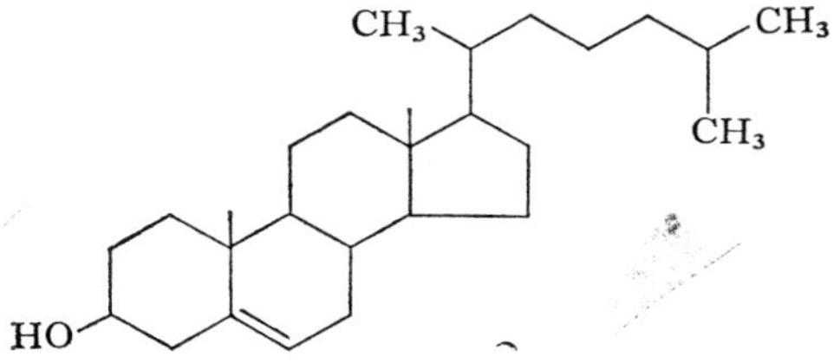

(15)

(15) did not produce anaesthesia in either sex. Selye noticed that with suitable doses, a quiet, deep, reversible anaesthesia could be produced without preliminary excitement. There was some peripheral vasodilatation. Death after high doses resulted from respiratory depression rather than from direct effects on the heart. He also found that partial hepatectomy but not bilateral nephrectomy increased the sensitivity to anaesthetic steroids, and concluded that the liver was important in their detoxification. Thus with his initial observations, Selye had established some of the important properties of steroid anaesthetics. He thought originally that only hormonally active steroids produced anaesthesia (Selye, 1941b) but subsequent work (Selye, 1942) showed that the most active compound he tested, 5β-pregnane-3,20-dione (16), was devoid of hormonal activity. Some of his conclusions on the relationship of structure to anaesthetic activity have not been substantiated by later work but he did warn against transferring one set of rules from one class of compounds to another.

6.3   FIRST CLINICAL USE OF STEROID ANAESTHESIA

No immediate practical use was made of Selye's findings. Merryman *et al.* (1954) produced sleep in women following the intravenous infusion of 200 or 500 mg of progesterone (11) dissolved in an albumin-propylene glycol mixture but the formulation was impracticable for widespread use.

Laubach *et al.* (1955) described the anaesthetic properties of hydroxydione (Viadril®) (17). It is the 21-hydroxy derivative of Selye's most active compound 5β-pregnane-3,20-dione (16) rendered water-soluble by esterification as the sodium hemisuccinate.

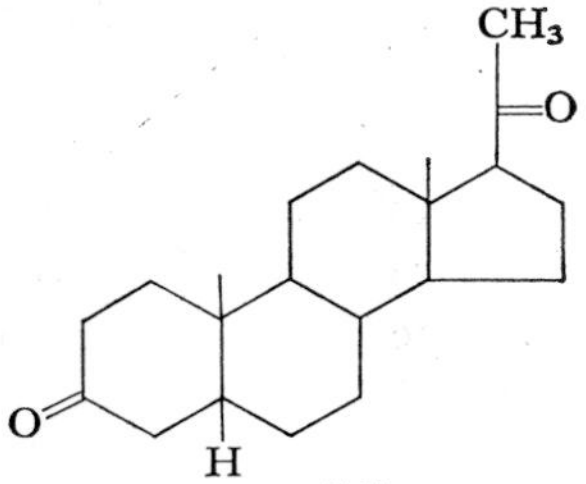

(16) 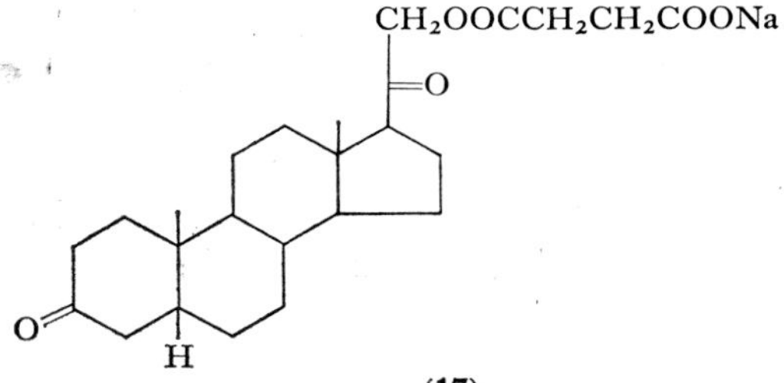   (17)

Hydroxydione produced a reversible depression of the central nervous system by the intravenous route in mice, rats, dogs and monkeys (P'an *et al.*, 1955). The onset of anaesthesia was smooth though delayed for several minutes, and recovery was rapid. There was a wide margin of safety. The first use of hydroxydione in man was reported by Gordan *et al.* (1955) and Murphy *et al.* (1955a). Extensive clinical experience (Dent *et al.*, 1956; Galley and Rooms, 1956; Laborit *et al.*, 1956) soon revealed a remarkable unanimity as to its properties. Induction was smooth and uncomplicated, beginning after 4 to 5 minutes but full anaesthesia was not achieved until 10 minutes after injection. The pharyngeal and laryngeal reflexes were depressed so that the airways could be intubated without the use of muscle-relaxants in some cases. Laryngospasm was rare but protective cough reflexes were still present so that the vocal cords contracted momentarily, if stimulated, and then relaxed. Full surgical anaesthesia was obtained only with large doses but there was no anti-analgesic action as seen with the rapidly acting barbiturates. In general, hydroxydione was regarded as a basal anaesthetic to be supplemented by analgesics or inhalational anaesthetics. Respiration was only slightly depressed, and there was some fall in blood pressure. The most commonly reported advantage of hydroxydione was the smooth uncomplicated recovery from anaesthesia. The incidence of nausea and vomiting was low, and post-operatively there was a feeling of general well-being amounting to euphoria in some cases.

Minor disadvantages of hydroxydione included the slowness of induction, the large dose required (0·5 to 1·5 g in man), occasional muscle twitches after induction, and the instability of the solution. The major disadvantages were pain on injection and a moderately high incidence of thrombophlebitis. Many attempts were made to overcome these two major problems either by using very dilute solutions given via a continuous drip (Murphy *et al.*, 1955b; Galley and Rooms, 1956) or by the injection of very concentrated solutions (Galley and Lerman, 1959). None was completely successful. Robertson and Wynn-Williams (1961) studied the pathology of the vein damage produced by hydroxydione. They considered that the pain and vein damage were not the result of the high pH of the hydroxydione solution but an inherent property of the molecule.

Despite its advantages as an anaesthetic, it was the tendency to cause venous irritation that curtailed the use of hydroxydione in the UK and the USA. Solutions of hydroxydione buffered with glycine for example (Primo and Lahon, 1965) are still in use in the continent of Europe.

6.4   STRUCTURE–ACTION RELATIONSHIPS

The selection of hydroxydione for clinical use was the culmination of the extensive screening programme described by Figdor *et al.* (1957). Selye's original findings provided the starting point for this work. The use of the intraperitoneal route in hepatectomized rats was abandoned as being unphysiological and too far removed from the anticipated mode of use of the anaesthetic. Subsequent work has confirmed that the intraperitoneal route is likely to provide information that is irrelevant when evaluating a drug for intravenous use, especially if the drug is rapidly metabolized in the liver. Figdor *et al.* (1957) chose the intravenous route in mice for screening purposes. To overcome the water-insolubility of most steroids, esters were prepared. Where these esters proved insoluble in water, or where the insoluble steroid was to be examined, solutions were made in dimethyl-acetamide, or suspensions were prepared using wetting agents. It was hoped that the soluble esters would be comparable pharmacologically with their parent compounds but this was true only in some respects. These authors found the hemisuccinate esters of nuclear unsaturated types such as desoxycorticosterone and progesterone disappointing, and their nuclear substituted homologues were inactive. They therefore turned to nuclear saturated types. A consideration of some stereochemically different pregnanes (3β, 5α; 3β, 5β and 3α, 5β) led to the conclusion that the differences between them were only minor and the importance of configuration was dismissed. However, it is probable that all had been reduced to a common mediocrity by esterification as hemisuccinates, and this may be why the authors ignored the superiority of compounds with a 3α-configuration (cf. compounds 1, 4 and 8 in their table 3). No mention was made at this stage of the speed of onset of anaesthesia, but delay in induction may explain why 3α-hydroxy-5β-pregnane-21-hemisuccinate sodium was not specifically commented upon though it appeared to have properties comparable with those of hydroxydione. It was recognized that saturated C-21 compounds substituted at 3 and 20 or 3, 20 and 21 appeared highly active, and that additional substitution was deleterious, often introducing stimulant properties. Though polarity and stereochemical factors were dismissed, the importance of the nature of the solubilizing group was recognized.

The speed of onset of anaesthesia was discussed for the first time when esters other than hemisuccinates were used for solubilization. Though anaesthetic potencies were often similar, the speed of onset varied over a three-fold range. Two factors influencing speed of onset were discussed. It was suggested that with the hemisuccinate esters speed of hydrolysis was the controlling factor, whereas the aminoacid esters, being weakly ionized in the blood, could pass into the central nervous system and act *per se* without preliminary hydrolysis to the parent alcohol. Rapid passage into the brain because of high lipid solubility was considered to explain the rapidity of onset, higher potency and greater toxicity of the amino esters, though rapid hydrolysis was not ruled out. Discussion of these factors led to consideration of the water-insoluble free alcohols, and the great rapidity of onset of the 3α-hydroxy compounds was noted. It was postulated that

TABLE 3

Induction and sleep times of steroids injected intravenously into male mice as solutions or suspensions in 20 per cent Cremophor EL

Formula	Form injected	Dose[a] mg kg^{-1}	Induction time[b] min	Sleep time[c] min
3α-Hydroxy-5α-pregnan-20-one	solution	3·1	1·4	8
3α-Hydroxy-5β-pregnan-20-one	solution	3·1	I	6
3β-Hydroxy-5α-pregnan-20-one	suspension	100	5 (4/5 only)	22
3β-Hydroxy-5β-pregnan-20-one	suspension	25	4	44
3α-Hydroxy-5α-pregnane-11,20-dione	solution	3·1	I	3·4
3α-Hydroxy-5β-pregnane-11,20-dione	solution	6·25	I	2
3β-Hydroxy-5α-pregnane-11,20-dione	suspension	50	5	35
3β-Hydroxy-5β-pregnane-11,20-dione	suspension	50	3·5	31

[a] Lowest dose producing loss of righting reflex in 5/5 mice.
[b] Time from end of injection to loss of righting reflex. I, immediate.
[c] Duration of loss of righting reflex.

the 3-ketones might become active only after metabolic reduction, but the results then available were thought insufficient for definitive conclusions.

Witzel (1959) in a review listed the published results of Selye (1941a, 1942) and Figdor et al. (1957), and the unpublished observations of Langecker and Busch on 26 weakly active steroids most of which were hemisuccinate esters. This paper added little to existing knowledge, as frequently comparisons were made between compounds in which more than one change had been made in the molecule. Kappas and Palmer (1963) reviewed existing knowledge.

P'an and Laubach (1964) re-examined their original conclusions (P'an et al., 1955; Figdor et al., 1957) on structure–activity relationships, and also gave an extensive description of the pharmacology of hydroxydione.

They suggested that anaesthetic activity was much less sensitive to structural detail than most other biological effects of steroids. This conclusion probably followed from the study of the relatively inactive ketones and water-soluble esters. They made the important observation that the structural requirements for high endocrine activity were not relevant to anaesthetic activity. The similar activity of the 5α and 5β series was found difficult to reconcile with a concept of receptor sites for the action of steroid anaesthetics. The importance of the configuration at the 3-position was ignored. Despite repeated emphasis on a lack of strict structural requirements for anaesthesia, it was pointed out that the possession of high lipid solubility was no guarantee that a steroid had central depressant effects. The authors did, however, predict that additional unpublished information might modify the apparent pattern of structure–function relationships. This review also discussed the absorption, distribution and metabolism of steroid anaesthetics.

Atkinson *et al.* (1965) had carried out a screening programme in the late 1950s with the object of producing a water-soluble anaesthetic with properties similar to hydroxydione but free of the tendency to cause thrombophlebitis. They tested 168 steroids by the intravenous route in mice either as solutions in 0·9 per cent sodium chloride or as suspensions in 0·4 per cent Tween 80. One hundred and forty-two were pregnane derivatives in either the 5α or 5β series. They included 3-keto, 3α or 3β-hydroxy 11-desoxy or 11-keto compounds tested as the free steroids, or their 3- or 21-hemisuccinate esters. A few other esters were examined. The most potent and rapidly acting compounds were those unesterified steroids with a free 3α-hydroxy group regardless of the configuration at carbon 5. Compounds with a 3-ketone group always produced a slower induction of anaesthesia than their 3α-hydroxy equivalents in the 5β series. The 3-ketones in the 5α series were generally inactive. The 3β-hydroxy-5α-pregnanes, either as free alcohols or as 3-hemisuccinate esters, were predominantly inactive, but the 11-keto derivatives of the 3-esters did show weak activity with slow induction. The presence of a free 21-hydroxy group conferred no advantage apart from providing a site for esterification to yield a water-soluble compound. The 11-keto compounds in the 5β series tended to be less active and less toxic, and induced anaesthesia more rapidly than their 11-unsubstituted analogues. Atkinson *et al.* (1965) selected 3α-hydroxy-5β-pregnane-11,20-dione 3-phosphate disodium (**18**) for clinical trial in man. It formed a stable aqueous solution, had a high margin of safety, was about two-thirds as potent as hydroxydione, and did not cause pain on injection or thrombophlebitis in animals. When examined in man, a dose of 1 to 1·5 g was required intravenously to produce sleep after a delay of about 5 minutes. Though free of venous irritant properties, it caused an unpleasant paraesthesia—a pins and needles sensation—extending over the head, trunk,

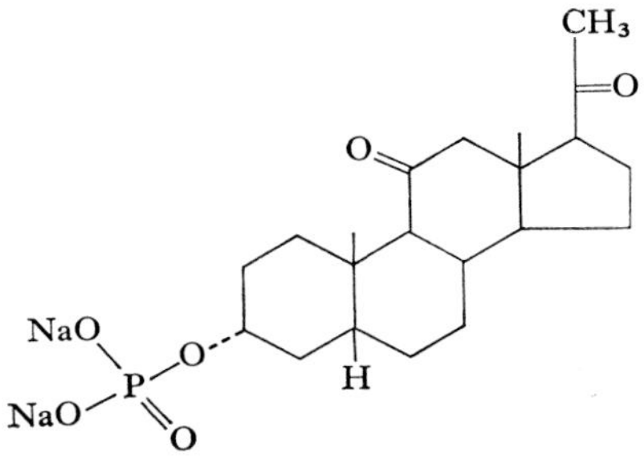

(18)

buttocks and legs. The effect started immediately after injection and lasted for a couple of minutes. Paraesthesia did not recur if further doses were given before consciousness was lost but the sensation experienced by the patient was too unpleasant to permit further use of this steroid.

Gyermek *et al.* (1968) summarized their work on 62 steroids some of which were new compounds. They were tested either in aqueous solution, dissolved in dimethyl sulphoxide or glycols, or suspended in carboxymethyl cellulose or Tween 20. They found 3α-hydroxy-5β-pregnan-20-one (19) to be the most potent compound by the intravenous route in mice, closely followed by 3α-hydroxy-18-methyl-5β-pregnan-20-one (20) and 3α-hydroxy-5β-pregnane-11,20-dione (21). They were more active when injected as solutions than as suspensions. The free alcohols with the 3α-configuration were the most potent, and esterification consistently reduced

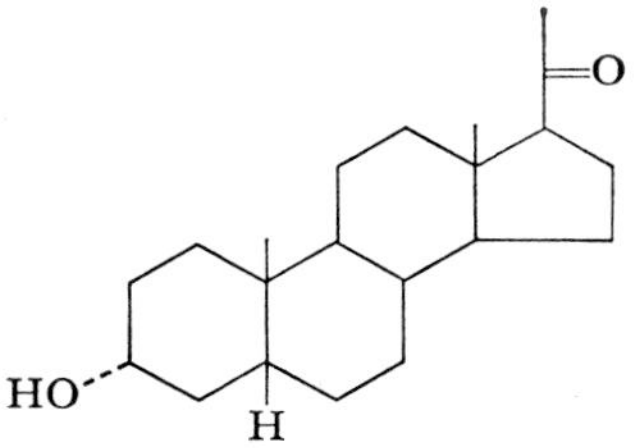

(19)

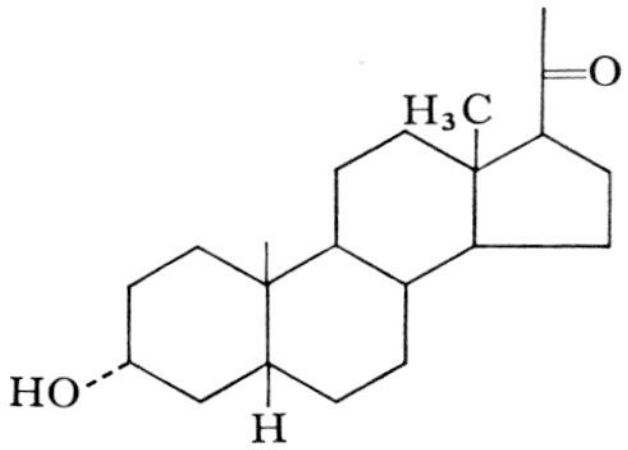

(20)

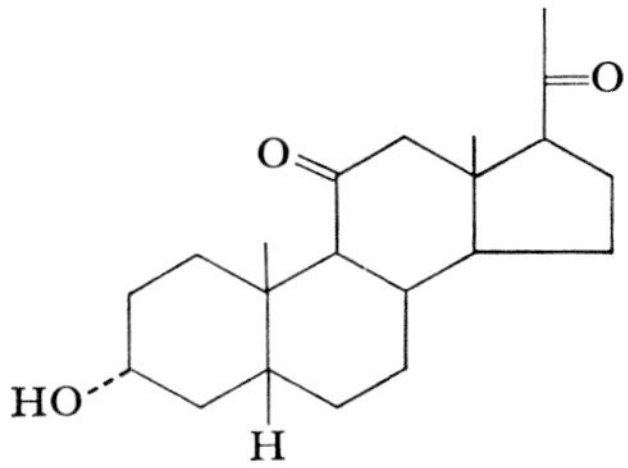

(21)

potency and slowed the onset of anaesthesia. Substituents other than 11-keto or 21-hydroxy when added to the C-3 and C-20 oxygen function interfered with anaesthetic potency. Though the pregn-4-enes and pregn-5-enes were described as less potent than the saturated pregnanes, these types were only tested in weakly active compounds such as 3β-hydroxy or 11β-hydroxy derivatives, so no general conclusions can be drawn from these findings. The 19-nor derivatives were as potent as their active 19-methyl equivalents.

The most active compound, 3α-hydroxy-5β-pregnan-20-one **(19)** (pregnanolone), was examined in a wide range of species and in various tests on the central nervous and cardiovascular systems of animals (Gyermek, 1967). As a naturally occurring metabolite of progesterone, the role of pregnanolone in the central nervous system was considered, and its relationship to the actions of the short-acting barbiturates on the brain was discussed tentatively. It was suggested that the findings gave further support to the view that the hypnotic actions of progesterone and sedation in pregnancy might be mediated through pregnanolone (Figdor et al., 1957).

6.5 DEVELOPMENT OF CT 1341

The Glaxo group returned to steroid anaesthetics in 1966 with new objectives. They sought a water-soluble steroid with the wide margin of safety, and the pleasant induction and recovery from anaesthesia found with hydroxydione. It should be free of the vascular irritant effects of hydroxydione and not cause the paraesthesia evoked by 3α-hydroxy-5β-pregnane-11,20-dione 3-phosphate disodium. In addition it should have the rapid induction and high potency of the rapidly-acting barbiturates. Such a compound would combine the advantages of hydroxydione and the barbiturates without some of their disadvantages.

From a consideration of structure–activity relationships it was clear that the type of compound likely to combine these properties could be found in the pregnanes of both the 5α and the 5β series if they possessed a free 3α-hydroxy group. An 11-keto group, though not essential, reduced toxicity and increased solubility in some instances. Table 3 compares the induction times and sleep times in mice of all the 3-hydroxy pregnanes in the 5α and 5β series either as the 20-ketones or as the 11,20 diketones. It will be seen that the 3α-hydroxy pregnanes were more potent and induced sleep more rapidly than their 3β-hydroxy analogues. Attempts to solubilize some of them as the 3- or 21-sodium hemisuccinates (Table 4) reduced potency and usually increased the induction time. It was clear that a compound combining most of the desirable properties was likely to be found among

TABLE 4

Induction and sleep times of steroid esters injected intravenously into male mice as aqueous solutions

Formula	Dose[a] mg kg^{-1}	Induction time[b] min	Sleep time[c] min
3α-Hydroxy-5β-pregnan-20-one 3-hemisuccinate sodium	30	3·2	22
3α-Hydroxy-5β-pregnane-11,20-dione 3-hemisuccinate sodium	40	3·2	10
3α, 21-Dihydroxy-5β-pregnane-11,20-dione 21-hemisuccinate sodium	175	6·7	19
3α-Hydroxy-5α-pregnane-11,20-dione 3-hemisuccinate sodium	100	7	14
3α,21-Dihydroxy-5α-pregnane-11,20-dione 21-hemisuccinate sodium	100	I	12

[a] Lowest dose producing loss of righting reflex in 5/5 mice.
[b] Time from end of injection to loss of righting reflex. I, immediate.
[c] Duration of loss of righting reflex.

the water-insoluble 3α-hydroxy pregnanes. Such a compound would be of use only if it could be dissolved in a biologically acceptable solvent for intravenous injection. Polyoxyethylated castor oil (Cremophor EL) was selected as it had been widely used in man to formulate the short-acting intravenous anaesthetic propanidid. The choice of the steroid lay between four compounds, 3α-hydroxy-5β-pregnan-20-one (19), 3α-hydroxy-5β-pregnane-11,20-dione (21), 3α-hydroxy-5α-pregnan-20-one (22), and 3α-hydroxy-5α-pregnane-11,20-dione (23). All had similar merits as anaesthetics in mice and the final selection rested on a combination of several factors. These included their propensity to provoke pyrexia, the speed of onset of anaesthesia and their solubility in Cremophor EL.

Pyrexia can follow the parenteral administration of certain steroids to man, and is usually greater after intramuscular than after intravenous injection. Regardless of the route of administration, there is a delay of 4 to 6 hours before the onset of pyrexia. The general features of steroid-induced pyrexia have been described by Kappas et al. (1959), Glickman et al. (1964), and reviewed by Kappas and Palmer (1965). The 5β-steroids tend to be more pyrogenic than the 5α-steroids (Kappas et al., 1957), so that (19) and (21) are particularly pyrogenic in man (Kappas et al., 1960). The exact mechanisms involved in steroid-induced pyrexia are unknown,

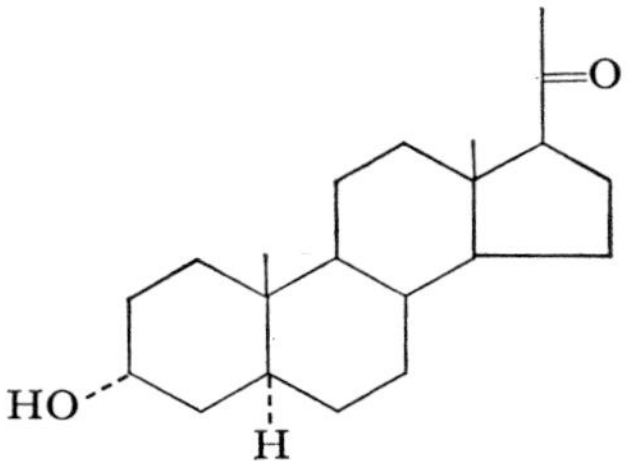

(22)

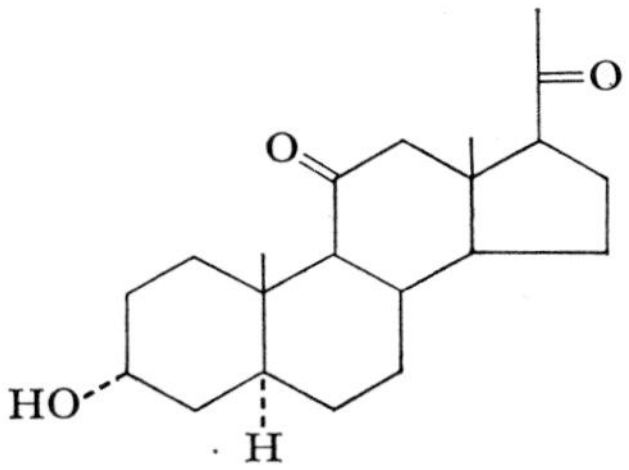

(23)

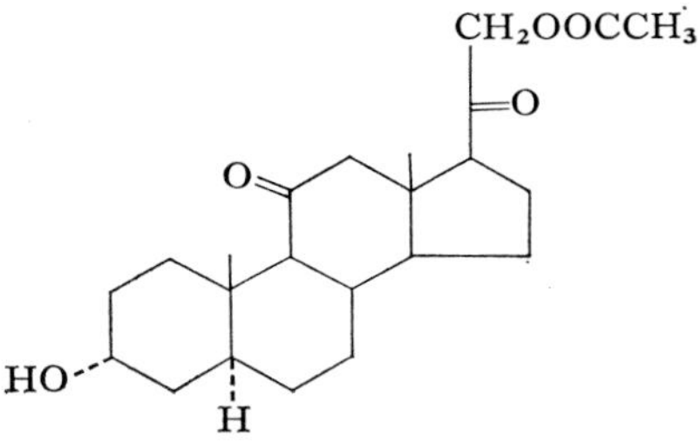

(24)

though recent work suggests that pyrogenic material is released from human but not from rabbit leucocytes (Bodel and Dillard, 1968).

A 5α-pregnane therefore seemed less likely to produce pyrexia in man than a 5β-pregnane. The 11-desoxy-5α-pregnan (22) did not produce rapid induction of anaesthesia and was not considered further. The 11-keto pregnanes (21) and (23) were both more soluble in Cremophor EL than their 11-desoxy equivalents (19) and (22) so the compound finally selected was 3α-hydroxy-5α-pregnane-11,20-dione (alphaxalone) (23). The solubility of alphaxalone was about 3 mg ml^{-1} in 20 per cent Cremophor EL but this could be increased at least three-fold if mixed with a small proportion of 21-acetoxy-3α-hydroxy-5α-pregnane-11,20-dione (alphadolone acetate) (24). Alphadolone acetate is half as potent as alphaxalone but has similar anaesthetic properties (Child *et al.*, 1971). A mixture of alphaxalone 9 mg ml^{-1} and alphadolone acetate 3 mg ml^{-1} in 20 per cent Cremophor EL containing 0·25 per cent sodium chloride was chosen for further examination under the name CT 1341 (Althesin® for human use, and Saffan® for veterinary use). Doses of CT 1341 are expressed in terms of the total steroid content (12 mg ml^{-1}) or the volume of solution.

6.5.1 *Pharmacology of CT 1341*

The pharmacological properties of CT 1341 in animals have been reported by Child *et al.* (1971, 1972a). The most unacceptable property of the original steroid anaesthetic hydroxydione was its tendency to cause thrombo-phlebitis. This is easily demonstrated by injecting mice via their tail veins with hydroxydione at a dose of 100 mg kg^{-1}. When examined 24 hours later the tails are blackish-blue and swollen, and may wither and drop off after a few days. The tails of mice injected with CT 1341 at a dose as high as 36 mg kg^{-1} show only a slight bruising at the injection site and are in-distinguishable from those injected with physiological saline. The deliberate injection of CT 1341 into the ear arteries of rabbits does not produce the severe necrosis that follows the intra-arterial injection of 5 per cent thio-pentone (Child *et al.*, 1971). This lack of vascular damage with CT 1341 has been confirmed in all species.

The wide margin of safety found with hydroxydione can also be demon-strated with CT 1341. The therapeutic index in mice (defined as the dose killing 50 per cent of animals (LD$_{50}$), divided by the dose causing 50 per cent of animals to lose their righting reflex (AD$_{50}$)) is 17·3 for hydroxydione and 30·6 for CT 1341 compared with 6·9, 7·4, 8·1 and 8·5 respectively for thiopentone, methohexitone, propanidid and ketamine (Child *et al.*, 1971). The therapeutic index expressed in this way exaggerates the practical safety margin but the relative proportions between the anaesthetics are confirmed in other species.

Unlike hydroxydione, induction of anaesthesia with CT 1341 is rapid in all species even at the lowest doses. Consciousness is lost within 15 to 30 seconds of the start of injection and presumably reflects the vein-to-brain circulation time. The minimum doses causing loss of righting reflex lie between 0·5 and 2 mg kg^{-1} for all species examined but the dose–activity response curves differ; the dog, cat and monkey are the most sensitive and the mouse is the least. Induction, sleep and recovery are uncomplicated in all species except the dog which shows an anaphylactoid reaction to the solvent Cremophor EL as described for propanidid. The cat was chosen for the major pharmacological study of CT 1341 preparatory to its assess-ment in man. This avoided the accumulation of results predominantly relevant to the dog only as occurred in the testing of propanidid.

In cats, CT 1341 produces anaesthesia over a wide range of doses. With 0·4 mg kg^{-1} there is only a loss of righting reflex lasting for about 1 minute and ataxia for 5 to 7 minutes. As the dose is raised, the depth and duration of anaesthesia increase. The corneal reflex is absent for about 3 minutes with 3·6 mg kg^{-1} and light surgical procedures are possible for 5 to 10 minutes with 7·2 mg kg^{-1}. The duration of effect can be extended by giving further doses as required. Deep surgical anaesthesia of 1 hour's duration follows a single dose of 19·2 mg kg^{-1} with only slight respiratory depression, but higher doses usually cause apnoea, vascular collapse and death unless ventilation is assisted. On recovery from anaesthesia, cats are eager to eat, and in the experimental situation no vomiting has been seen.

In mice, repeated doses of CT 1341 are almost noncumulative in marked contrast to thiopentone (Child *et al.*, 1971). This is also the case in cats kept in a state of surgical anaesthesia for 3 hours with repeated intravenous doses of CT 1341 or thiopentone. The cats were fully recovered 2 hours after the last dose of CT 1341 but were not behaviourally normal until 48 hours after the last dose of thiopentone (Dodds and Twissell, 1973).

The anaesthetic, cardiovascular, respiratory, and adverse effects of CT 1341, thiopentone, methohexitone, propanidid and ketamine have been compared in unrestrained cats fitted with permanently indwelling intra-venous and intra-arterial cannulae (Child *et al.*, 1972a). CT 1341 could be administered intravenously over a range of 5 doubling doses (1·2 to 19·2 mg kg^{-1}) with only slight respiratory depression at the top dose, whereas thiopentone and methohexitone caused definite respiratory depression at the top 2 of 4 doubling doses (3 to 24 mg kg^{-1}). Surgical anaesthesia was not achieved with propanidid in the cat. Ketamine provided good surgical conditions with analgesia though respiration was severely depressed at the top doses, recovery was slow and there were many adverse effects. The cardiovascular effects of CT 1341 and thiopentone were similar in the cat at comparable anaesthetic doses. There was an initial tachycardia and fall in blood pressure at the higher doses. Adverse effects such as flushing, defaecation and emergence excitement occurred randomly with all the anaesthetics but were seen least with CT 1341 and thiopentone. Oedema of the paws and ears was seen in some cats after CT 1341 and passed off uneventfully within an hour. The incidence was variable, some cats showed the effect after each injection, others not at all. Cats showing this reaction exhibited no different anaesthetic or cardiovascular response to CT 1341 than those not reacting. The effect was attributable to the vehicle for the steroids, Cremophor EL.

In experiments designed to simulate the use of CT 1341 in anaesthetic practice, CT 1341 was completely acceptable when used alone or after pre-medicants, or used in conjunction with anaesthetic adjuvants, neuro-muscular blocking agents and inhalational anaesthetics (Child *et al.*, 1971). The usually trivial respiratory depressant effects of CT 1341 were potentiated when CT 1341 was administered during full anaesthesia with other anaesthetics, particularly the barbiturates and α-chloralose (Child *et al.*, 1972a). This interaction is similar to that reported between hydroxy-dione and α-chloralose (Lerman and Paton, 1960).

CT 1341 is almost devoid of hormonal activity. It is inactive in tests for oestrogenic, progestational and mineralocorticoid activity but does show weak anti-uterotropic activity (Child *et al.*, 1972b). The weak thymolytic activity originally reported (Child *et al.*, 1971) has not been confirmed in subsequent tests. CT 1341 has no adverse effect on the growth and fertility of mice when administered before mating or throughout pregnancy. It did not cause premature parturition in mice and rats when given in large, near lethal doses at the end of pregnancy, and the offspring of all animals dosed with CT 1341 grew normally and proved fertile (Child *et al.*, 1972b). Similar results have been obtained in rabbits dosed throughout or at the end of pregnancy (Gilbert *et al.*, 1973).

6.5.2   *Clinical use of CT 1341 in animals*

Evans *et al.* (1972) described the first clinical use of CT 1341 in cats by the intravenous or intramuscular routes. They concluded that a dose of 0·75 ml kg^{-1} (9 mg kg^{-1}) intravenously, rapidly induces anaesthesia lasting 10 to 12 minutes sufficient for castration or dental procedures. The required level of anaesthesia could be maintained for longer periods with small supplementary doses of CT 1341 as required. The results with CT 1341 by the intramuscular route were variable. Some veterinary surgeons found it completely satisfactory in all cases whilst others found that it did not produce the required degree of sedation or was completely ineffective. These results suggested that the method of intramuscular administration employed by different individuals was influencing the results. It seemed likely that the inadvertent injection of part or all of the dose into the fascial planes instead of into muscle could result in slow absorption. Such a situation, combined with the rapid elimination of CT 1341, would mean that effective anaesthetic concentrations were not achieved in the brain. When an intramuscular injection technique was adopted which ensured deep intramuscular injection into the quadriceps, the success rate increased considerably. It is perhaps interesting to speculate how often other drugs injected by the intramuscular route are inadvertently deposited in the fascia. The rapid onset and short duration of action of CT 1341 revealed this possibility and it was confirmed by injecting coloured solutions. Following injection into the lateral aspect of the cat's thigh, the majority of the solution was found to lie along the connective tissue around the sciatic nerve in a high proportion of cases (Baxter and Evans, 1973).

Hall (1972) reported results in 71 cats and included preliminary observations in horses, sheep and pigs. He found that 0·5 ml kg^{-1} (6 mg kg^{-1}) of CT 1341 intravenously in cats could be used as the sole anaesthetic for procedures lasting up to 20 minutes. Anaesthesia could then be maintained with incremental doses one-third to one-half the original dose. There were small falls in blood pressure accompanied by an increase in heart rate but respiratory rate was unchanged. No changes were seen in the electrocardiogram. After induction with CT 1341, anaesthesia could be maintained with nitrous oxide, halothane, methoxyflurane or ether, and intubation could be facilitated with suxamethonium. Side effects included sneezing, and skin hyperaemia of the nose, ear pinnae and paws. Oedematous swelling of the interdigital web was seen in one cat. Two cats retched during induction but otherwise induction of anaesthesia was smooth, rapid and uneventful. Surgical conditions were excellent, and recovery from anaesthesia was reasonably rapid though commonly accompanied by muscle twitching. Surgical anaesthesia developed 7 to 10 minutes after an intramuscular dose of 15 to 18 mg kg^{-1}, and the injection of the relatively large volume was apparently painless and left no residual effects.

In initial trials, horses required a minimum intravenous dose of 1·2 mg kg^{-1}. Recovery was complicated by emergence excitement but this could be diminished by pretreatment with acepromazine, or abolished with xylazine, though this delayed recovery. In sheep, CT 1341 consistently produced bradycardia, a decrease in blood pressure, and a decrease in cardiac output for several minutes after each dose. CT 1341 prevented suxamethonium-induced hyperpyrexia in susceptible Landrace pigs and did not itself produce hyperpyrexia in these animals. These preliminary findings in pigs have been confirmed in further experiments by Hall et al. (1972). Harrison (1973), however, showed that whilst CT 1341 blocked halothane-induced hyperpyrexia in pigs it had no effect on the established syndrome and did not prevent the initiation of hyperpyrexia by suxamethonium. Clearly there must be differences in technique or in the strain of animals used.

6.5.3 Clinical use of CT 1341 in man

The first clinical trial of CT 1341 involved 20 patients (Campbell et al., 1971). In a pilot experiment 8 patients were given doses in the range 3 to 10 ml (0·05 to 1·7 mg kg^{-1}) predicted from animal experiments (the upper dose being equivalent to the AD_{50} dose in mice). Induction was rapid (30 to 80 seconds) though slightly longer than with thiopentone. No apnoea, respiratory depression, laryngospasm or bronchospasm occurred, the ECG pattern was normal and there was a rise in heart rate. There appeared to be a trivial rise in blood pressure but a definite peripheral vasodilatation was seen as a flushing of the skin. Some patients showed muscle movement and tremor after induction. Recovery was rapid, within 15 to 360 seconds of the end of any inhalational anaesthetic. Most patients had a feeling of euphoria—an effect also reported after hydroxydione.

There was no pain, irritation at the injection site or vein damage. The next 6 patients, who were catheterized for the diagnosis of heart conditions, received a standardized dose of 1·2 mg kg^{-1}. The results were similar to those of the pilot experiment but with some additions and exceptions. Direct measurement of blood pressure showed falls of up to 20 per cent beginning 30 seconds after injection but there was no significant fall in cardiac output. The arterial P_{aO_2} showed a significant fall and the P_{aCO_2} showed a slight rise. The respiratory rate was increased, and pupils were dilated. There was no nausea or vomiting. The first clinical trial was completed with a study of recovery time in 6 patients given a dose of 1·8 mg kg^{-1} supplemented with nitrous oxide. Recovery was considered complete when patients were able to stand unassisted with their eyes closed (negative Rombergism). Recovery time for CT 1341 (24 minutes) was similar to that for methohexitone (25 minutes) and thiopentone (28 minutes) but longer than after propanidid (18 minutes). The clinical trial was then extended to several centres. Bradford et al. (1971) used CT 1341 in conjunction with anaesthetic adjuvants and inhalational anaesthetics. There were no interactions with suxamethonium, (+)-tubocurarine or pancuronium, or with halothane or trilene but there was a marked sinus tachycardia with methoxyflurane. A practical dose–response regimen was established in 300 patients undergoing minor gynaecological surgery (Clarke et al., 1971). The term μl was adopted for expressing the induction doses which ranged from 25 to 200 μl kg^{-1} (equivalent to 0·3 to 2·4 mg kg^{-1}). The CT 1341 was supplemented with nitrous oxide 75 per cent oxygen 25 per cent or 100 μl doses of CT 1341 where necessary. A dose range of 40 to 100 μl kg^{-1} was found acceptable with 50 to 60 μl kg^{-1} providing optimum surgical conditions with least side effects. Patients lost consciousness in one arm-to-brain circulation time. Involuntary muscle movement soon after injection was greater with the higher doses but subsided spontaneously. The incidence was higher than with thiopentone but less than with methohexitone. Respiration was not depressed except at the highest doses (200 μl kg^{-1}). Falls in blood pressure were mainly in the range 0 to 20 mmHg, and the incidence of significant hypotension increased with dose. There were no instances of falls of 60 mmHg or more even with the 200 μl kg^{-1} dose. Recovery was rapid, most patients wakening within 2 minutes of the cessation of the inhalational anaesthetic when given the optimum dose of CT 1341. The incidence of nausea and vomiting was lower than previously reported for thiopentone, methohexitone, propanidid or ketamine. Though the euphoria mentioned by Campbell et al. (1971) was not found, over 90 per cent of patients liked anaesthesia with CT 1341. Savege et al. (1971) studied the cardiovascular effects of standard doses of 50 and 100 μl kg^{-1} of CT 1341 in 23 fit subjects fitted with indwelling arterial and venous cannulae. Induction was smooth and rapid, and in general their results agreed with those of Campbell *et al.* (1971). They found falls in blood pressure of up to 24 per cent and an increase in heart rate but cardiac output was sustained despite a marked fall in central venous pressure. Swerdlow *et al.* (1971) used CT 1341 as the sole anaesthetic in single or repeated doses in 109 patients or supplemented with nitrous oxide and oxygen in a further 44 patients. Their results were in general agreement with those of earlier workers and they commented particularly on the rapid recovery, low incidence of nausea and vomiting, and lack of local irritation. Salivation and pupillary dilatation occurred in some of these unpremedicated patients.

The use of CT 1341 in many different situations was reported at a symposium in London in January 1972. Particular aspects not covered in earlier publications included a group trial on 800 patients conducted by 20 anaesthetists (Carson, 1972), electroconvulsive therapy (Foley *et al.*, 1972), intra-occular surgery (Fordham *et al.*, 1972), dentistry (Warren, 1972), and poor-risk patients (Miller *et al.*, 1972a).

6.5.4 *Metabolism and elimination of CT 1341*

The lack of cumulative effect with CT 1341 suggested that the steroids are rapidly inactivated or eliminated from the body. Autoradiographic studies in rats using ^{14}C-labelled steroids showed that alphaxalone and alphadolone acetate or their metabolites are concentrated in the liver and kidneys within minutes of intravenous injection and excreted in the bile and urine. In pregnant rats, small quantities of radioactivity reached the foetuses where distribution was similar to that seen in the mother (Card *et al.*, 1972). The steroids are excreted in the bile of rats predominantly as highly polar, conjugated, inactive metabolites, and 76 per cent of the radioactive dose of ^{14}C-labelled alphaxalone was recovered from the cannulated bile duct within 3 hours. Radiochromatographic studies of the bile indicated that conjugated 2α-hydroxy-alphaxalone is probably the major metabolite in the rat. The half-life of alphaxalone in rat plasma is approximately 7 minutes when assayed by a gas–liquid chromatography technique but longer when measurements of plasma radioactivity are made, suggesting the presence of circulating, possibly re-absorbed, metabolites (Child *et al.*, 1972c). Preliminary studies of rat urine indicate the presence of conjugated 2α,16α-dihydroxy-alphaxalone. This metabolite has not been detected in human urine where the major metabolites are 20-hydroxy-alphaxalone and 21-hydroxyalphaxalone. In the cat the plasma half-life of alphaxalone is 3 to 4 minutes and inactive metabolites appear rapidly in the bile but their exact nature has not been established so far (Gibson, unpublished results).

6.5.5 *Conclusions on CT 1341*

CT 1341 is now in use in many countries. Recent reports on its use tend to duplicate the findings of earlier workers though details are influenced by particular situations. The exact place of CT 1341 in anaesthesia is not yet established but includes its use as an induction agent and as the sole anaesthetic, as well as special applications. For example, CT 1341 lowers intracranial pressure in animals and man. It is therefore a suitable anaesthetic in patients with intracranial compression and in neurosurgical procedures (Pickerodt *et al.*, 1972; Turner *et al.*, 1973; Takahashi *et al.*, 1973). CT 1341 has been used successfully in one patient known to develop malignant hyperpyrexia after other anaesthetics (Isaacs and Barlow, 1973).

Some general conclusions can be drawn about the properties of CT 1341. It has overcome some minor and major deficiencies of the first steroid anaesthetic hydroxydione, namely slowness in inducing anaesthesia, low potency, pain on injection, and vascular irritancy. The advantages claimed for hydroxydione—a wide safety margin, little respiratory depression, smooth uncomplicated recovery from anaesthesia, and a low incidence of post-operative nausea and vomiting—have been retained. In addition there is very little cumulation of action with repeated doses and no cases of simple pyrexia or malignant hyperpyrexia have been reported. CT 1341 and hydroxydione lack definite analgesic action and share some unwanted side actions. Arora *et al.* (1972) in an experimental study with CT 1341 demonstrated slight anti-analgesic actions but these were less than those previously reported for thiopentone and were considered unlikely to be of great clinical significance. Most clinicians have seen varying degrees of muscle movement and twitching though less than after methohexitone. Tachycardia and falls in blood pressure comparable with those seen following thiopentone have been commented upon frequently but there is no agreement as to their clinical significance. There have been a number of reports of sensitivity reactions to CT 1341 (Austin *et al.*, 1973; Avery and Evans, 1973; Hester, 1973; Horton, 1973; Mehta, 1973; Notcutt, 1973; Dundee *et al.*, 1974). Whether the incidence is greater than for other intravenous anaesthetics or reflects the reporting of results for a new drug is uncertain. Dundee and Clarke (1973) have offered to collate reports of suspected idiosyncrasy to all intravenous anaesthetics in the hope of clarifying the position.

CT 1341 represents a definite advance on hydroxydione but still does not fulfil all the criteria for the ideal intravenous anaesthetic suggested in the introduction.

7 The objectives and testing of intravenous anaesthetics

The major objective is to produce water-soluble compounds that are sufficiently lipid soluble to pass rapidly into the brain and are then rapidly eliminated. Combination of the first two seemingly incompatible properties has been achieved by adopting two different expedients both of which can introduce undesirable consequences. With propanidid and CT 1341, the surface–active agent Cremophor EL has been used to form water-miscible solutions. The amount of active compound that can be dissolved by Cremophor EL is relatively small and this limits the dose that can be given, particularly to large animals or by the intramuscular route. Further, the presence of Cremophor EL precludes use in dogs, and also provides a putative culprit for any untoward reaction seen in patients during anaesthesia. With the rapidly acting barbiturates and with hydroxydione, aqueous solutions are achieved by using sodium salts at a high pH. Though high pH may not be directly responsible for the tissue irritation that can be produced by barbiturate solutions, the momentary precipitation of the barbiturate that occurs as the solution approaches the pH of the blood probably plays some part in the necrosis that follows accidental arterial injection of barbiturates. Apart from the tendency to cause vascular damage, hydroxydione suffers from two other major deficiencies: slow induction and low potency. These properties could result from one or all of three factors. First, being a highly ionized compound, only the nonionized lipid-soluble fraction can cross the blood-brain barrier. Second, hydrolysis of the ester might be necessary before the steroid can enter the brain in an active form. Third, as the speed of onset of a 3-ketone is always slower than that of a 3α-hydroxy steroid it is probable that hydroxydione has to be reduced to the 3-hydroxy form to be active. P'an and Laubach (1964) when speculating on the form in which hydroxydione was active, favoured ester hydrolysis as the essential precursor of anaesthetic activity. They barely mentioned the influence of ionization, and ignored the effect of the 3-ketone. If the degree of ionization were the only factor operating one would expect reduced potency but the speed of onset would not necessarily be delayed. The rate of ester hydrolysis and reduction of the 3-ketone are both factors which slow induction. All three factors—ionization, ester hydrolysis and ketone reduction—reduce potency if metabolic inactivation is occurring concurrently.

All evidence obtained so far confirms the original prediction by Selye (1941a) that the duration of action of steroid anaesthetics is governed by metabolism, rather than by redistribution. Presumably, inactivation of a highly potent, rapidly acting steroid of short duration is well within the metabolic capacity of the liver, and probably accounts for the high therapeutic index and lack of cumulation with this type of anaesthetic. The therapeutic dose is determined by the proportion passing to the brain and that inactivated during passage through the liver on each circulation. Solubilization of a compound by the formation of a highly ionized salt. though perfectly acceptable with slow-acting, slowly metabolized anti-inflammatory steroids for example, is clearly inappropriate for a rapidly acting anaesthetic steroid of short duration. Any future water-soluble steroid anaesthetic, to be rapidly acting and potent, would have to be weakly ionized at blood pH. This may be difficult to achieve.

By contrast, the duration of action of rapidly acting barbiturates is governed by redistribution into depot tissues. Here the therapeutic dose initially is one which is sufficient to affect the brain as well as passing into other tissues. As the barbiturate redistributes from the brain into depot tissues anaesthesia lightens. Metabolism occurs relatively slowly and mostly provides the mechanism whereby the barbiturate is eventually eliminated from the body. As can be deduced from experiments where repeated doses of barbiturates are given, the depot tissues are soon saturated. The proportion of the dose available in the circulation to pass into the brain and other susceptible tissues increases dramatically and the barbiturate is no longer short acting. Thus future barbiturates will show less tendency to cumulate only if their duration of action is governed more by metabolism than by redistribution.

The introduction of propanidid and CT 1341 has demonstrated that rapidly acting anaesthetics of short duration can be found among compounds with structures other than the barbiturates, though the methods of solubilization used so far have introduced new problems.

Etomidate, R-(+)-ethyl 1-(α-methylbenzyl)imidazole-5-carboxylate, (R 16659) (25) is another new structural type producing rapid onset of anaesthesia of short duration (Janssen et al., 1971). This compound is currently undergoing clinical evaluation. Preliminary results suggest that it produces little depression of respiration or disturbance of circulation, and no unpleasant subjective impressions (Doenicke et al., 1973a, 1973b). Further, it releases less histamine into the blood plasma than other intravenous anaesthetics (Doenicke et al., 1973c).

(25)

Phencyclidine and ketamine provide a new class of anaesthetics producing what is termed dissociative anaesthesia. Here the speed of onset is slightly slower, the duration of action tends to be longer, and the quality of anaesthesia differs from conventional anaesthetics. Etoxadrol (CL-1848C), the dextrorotatory isomer of 2-ethyl-2-phenyl-4-(2-piperidyl)-(1,3-dioxolane hydrochloride) (26), is claimed to produce dissociative anaesthesia though it has little chemical similarity to ketamine (Traber et al., 1970; Wilson et al., 1970; Hidalgo et al., 1971). Etoxadrol is more potent than ketamine though of similar duration, but it is not yet clear if it is free of the psychic effects seen with phencyclidine and ketamine.

(26)

In many ways the initial screening of injectable anaesthetics should be relatively straightforward. The extent to which structure, potency and mode of elimination of a compound influence its properties depends on the route of administration. Selye was using the intraperitoneal route when he first demonstrated the comparatively weak anaesthetic activity of certain steroids. With the highly active compounds, the intraperitoneal route is inappropriate. It is probable that a large proportion of the dose is absorbed via the hepatic portal system, and rapidly inactivated in the liver. Only that proportion which is absorbed by other routes, or overloads the metabolic capacity of the liver, can reach the brain. To reduce metabolic inactivation by partial hepatectomy only confuses the situation. One consequence of the use of the intraperitoneal route is the difference in sensitivity to steroid anaesthetics shown by male and female rats described by Selye (1941a). This type of difference in sensitivity is sometimes seen in rats with slowly metabolized compounds, particularly if the oral or intraperitoneal routes are used, but is much less common in other species (Weston Hurst, 1958; Busfield et al., 1960). CT 1341 is more potent in female than in male rats by the oral route, and very large doses are required to produce sleep in either sex (Hart, unpublished observation). There is no sex difference in rats given normal doses of CT 1341 by the intravenous route (Child et al., 1971). The difference in sensitivity according to the route of administration probably reflects the well-known difference in metabolic capacity between male and female rats (Gram and Gillette, 1971). It only becomes apparent when doses are used which overload the metabolic capacity of the female rat liver.

For screening purposes, the most practical way to reduce the effects of inactivation by the liver is to inject the anaesthetic by the intravenous route. A steroid can be administered as a fine suspension or in a water-miscible solvent. For reasons already discussed, it must not be assumed that a water-soluble derivative has properties similar to its water-insoluble analogue. Administration of anaesthetics by the intravenous route in mice gives information on the speed of induction, potency, duration of action, the dose–response curve, and lethality, as well as evidence of pain or local tissue damage. Atkinson et al. (1965), when testing a series of anaesthetic steroids, chose the dose producing loss of righting reflex for 25 minutes in mice as their criterion for activity. This "25-minute sleeptime" dose was selected as many of the compounds tested produced slow induction, and with "15-minute sleeptime" doses or less, some animals did not lose their righting reflex. This was probably a mistaken choice as the AD_{50} dose in mice gives a better prediction of the anaesthetic activity of both hydroxydione and CT 1341 in man. The AD_{50} dose for hydroxydione in mice is 21·5 mg kg^{-1} (Laubach et al., 1955) whilst the generally accepted clinical dose range in man is 0·5 to 1·5 g, equivalent to 7 to 21 mg kg^{-1}. Similarly the AD_{50} dose for CT 1341 is 1·8 mg kg^{-1} (Child et al., 1971) and the dose range in man is about 0·5 to 1·8 mg kg^{-1} (Campbell et al., 1971; Clarke et al., 1971). Thus with the slowly acting, weakly potent hydroxydione, and with the rapidly acting, highly potent CT 1341, the mouse AD_{50} dose predicts the upper end of the dose range in man. However, with the barbiturates propanidid and ketamine, the mouse AD_{50} dose overestimates the human dose and must be interpreted with caution.

Once a compound has been selected from the initial screening procedure in mice, its anaesthetic and pharmacodynamic profile must be assessed in a variety of species. Despite subtle variations in response in particular animal tests, the broad properties of an anaesthetic can be established before its first use in man. Animal tests cannot conclusively predict all the properties of an anaesthetic, especially psychic effects, but careful study of the behaviour of animals can indicate where problems might arise.

As stated earlier, most anaesthetics succeed or fail as a result of their properties which are additional to those producing anaesthesia. Anaesthetics have profound effects on every system of the body, and it is the study of these effects which makes the topic of anaesthesia so fascinating. Interest in noninhalational anaesthetics is increasing at present as exemplified by the publication of a monograph devoted exclusively to intravenous anaesthesia (Dundee and Wyant, 1974). With our increasing understanding of the factors which produce the good and bad properties of an anaesthetic, we are now nearer to producing the ideal anaesthetic.

References

Anderson, N. B. and Amaranath, L. (1973). *Anesthesiology*, **39**, 126.

Arora, M. V., Carson, I. W. and Dundee, J. W. (1972). *British Journal of Anaesthesia*, **44**, 590.

Atkinson, R. M., Davis, B., Pratt, M. A., Sharpe, H. M. and Tomich, E. G. (1965). *Journal of Medicinal Chemistry* **8**, 426.

Austin, T. R., Anderson, J. and Richardson, J. (1973). *British Medical Journal*, **ii**, 661.

Avery, A. F. and Evans, A. (1973). *British Journal of Anaesthesia*, **45**, 301.

Barry, C. T., Lawson, R. and Davidson, D. G. D. (1967). *Anaesthesia*, **22**, 228.

Baxter, J. S. and Evans, J. M. (1973). *Journal of Small Animal Practice*, **14**, 297.

Beer, R. and Soga, D. (1971). *Anaesthesist*, **20**, 480.

Bernhoff, A., Eklund, B. and Kaijser, L. (1972). *British Journal of Anaesthesia*, **44**, 2.

Black, J. W., Duncan, W. A. M., Durant, C. J., Ganellin, C. R. and Parsons, E. M. (1972). *Nature*, **236**, 385.

Bodel, P. and Dillard, M. (1968). *Journal of Clinical Investigation*, **47**, 107.

Bradford, E. M. W., Miller, D. C., Campbell, D. and Baird, W. L. M. (1971). *British Journal of Anaesthesia*, **43**, 940.

Brand, L., Mark, L. C., Snell, M. M., Vrindten, P. and Dayton, P. G. (1963). *Anesthesiology*, **24**, 331.

Brodie, B. B., Mark, L. C., Papper, E. M., Lief, P. A., Bernstein, E. and Rovenstine, E. A. (1950). *Journal of Pharmacology and Experimental Therapeutics*, **98**, 85.

Brodie, B. B., Bernstein, E. and Mark, L. C. (1952). *Journal of Pharmacology and Experimental Therapeutics*, **105**, 421.

Brown, S. S., Lyons, S. M. and Dundee, J. W. (1968). *British Journal of Anaesthesia*, **40**, 13.

Busfield, D., Child, K. J., Basil, B. and Tomich, E. G. (1960). *Journal of Pharmacy and Pharmacology*, **12**, 539.

Bush, M. T. (1961). *Microchemistry Journal*, **5**, 73.

Bush, M. T. (1963). *In* "Physiological Pharmacology" (Eds W. S. Root and F. G. Hofmann) vol. 1, p. 205. Academic Press, New York and London.

Campbell, D., Forrester, A. C., Miller, D. C., Hutton, I., Kennedy, J. A., Lawrie, T. D. V., Lorimer, A. R. and McCall, D. (1971). *British Journal of Anaesthesia*, **43**, 14.

Card, B., McCulloch, R. J. and Pratt, D. A. H. (1972). *Postgraduate Medical Journal* **48**, Supplement (2), 34.

Carson, I. W. (1972). *Postgraduate Medical Journal* **48**, Supplement (2), 108.

Carson, I. W., Moore, J., Balmer, J. P., Dundee, J. W. and McNabb, T. G. (1973). *Anesthesiology*, **38**, 128.

Chang, T. and Glazko, A. J. (1972). *Anesthesiology*, **36**, 401.

Chang, T., Dill, W. A. and Glazko, A. J. (1965). *Federation Proceedings*, **24**, 268.

Chang, T., Savory, A., Albin, M., Goulet, R. and Glazko, A. J. (1970). *Clinical Research* **18**, 597.

Chen, G. M. and Weston, J. K. (1960). *Anesthesia and Analgesia (Cleveland)*, *Current Researches*, **39**, 132.

Chen, G., Ensor, C. R., Russell, D. and Bohner, B. (1959). *Journal of Pharmacology and Experimental Therapeutics*, **127**, 241.

Child, K. J., Currie, J. P., Davis, B., Dodds, M. G., Pearce, D. R. and Twissell, D. J. (1971). *British Journal of Anaesthesia*, **43**, 2.

Child, K. J., Davis, B., Dodds, M. G. and Twissell, D. J. (1972a). *British Journal of Pharmacology*, **46**, 189.

Child, K. J., English, A. F., Gilbert, H. G. and Woollett, E. A. (1972b). *Postgraduate Medical Journal*, **48**, Supplement (2), 51.

Child, K. J., Gibson, W., Harnby, G. and Hart, J. W. (1972c). *Postgraduate Medical Journal*, **48**, Supplement (2), 37.

Clarke, R. S. J. (1968). *British Journal of Anaesthesia*, **40**, 781.

Clarke, R. S. J. (1969). *International Anesthesiology Clinics*, **7**, 43.

Clarke, R. S. J. and Dundee, J. W. (1966). *British Journal of Anaesthesia*, **38**, 401.

Clarke, R. S. J., Dundee, J. W. and Hamilton, R. C. (1967). *Anaesthesia*, **22**, 235.

Clarke, R. S. J., Dundee, J. W., Barron, D. W. and McArdle, L. (1968). *British Journal of Anaesthesia*, **40**, 593.

Clarke, R. S. J., Montgomery, S. J., Dundee, J. W. and Bovill, J. G. (1971). *British Journal of Anaesthesia*, **43**, 947.

Clutton-Brock, J. C. (1960). *Anaesthesia*, **15**, 71.

Cohen, S. M. (1948a). *Lancet*, **ii**, 361.

Cohen, S. M. (1948b). *Lancet*, **ii**, 409.

Cohen, M. L., Chan, S.-L., Way, W. L. and Trevor, A. J. (1973). *Anesthesiology*, **39**, 370.

Collier, B. B. (1972). *Anaesthesia*, **27**, 120.

Conway, C. M., Ellis, D. B. and King, N. W. (1968). *British Journal of Anaesthesia*, **40**, 736.

Corssen, G. (1964). *International Anesthesiology Clinics*, **2**, 773.

Corssen, G. and Domino, E. F. (1966). *Anesthesia and Analgesia (Cleveland)*, *Current Researches*, **45**, 29.

Corssen, G., Miyasaka, M. and Domino, E. F. (1968). *Anesthesia and Analgesia (Cleveland)*, *Current Researches*, **47**, 746.

Dayton, P. G., Perel, J. M., Landrau, M. A., Brand, L. and Mark, L. C. (1967). *Biochemical Pharmacology*, **16**, 2321.

Dean, G. (1969). *South African Medical Journal*, **43**, 227.

Dent, S. J., Wilson, W. P. and Stephen, C. R. (1956). *Anesthesiology*, **17**, 672.

Dill, W. A., Chucot, L., Chang, T. and Glazko, A. J. (1971). *Anesthesiology*, **34**, 73.

Dodds, M. G. and Twissell, D. J. (1973). *Journal of Small Animal Practice*, **14**, 487.

Doenicke, A., Gürtner, T., Kugler, J., Schellenberger, A. and Spiess, W. (1965). *Anaesthesiologie und Wiederbelebung*, **4**, 249.

Doenicke, A., Krumey, I., Kugler, J. and Klempa, J. (1968). *British Journal of Anaesthesia*, **40**, 415.

Doenicke, A., Kugler, J., Penzel, G., Laub, M., Kalmar, L., Killian, I. and Bezecny, H. (1973a). *Anaesthesist*, **22**, 357.

Doenicke, A., Lorenz, W., Beigl, R., Bezecny, H., Uhlig, R., Kalmar, L., Praetorius, B. and Mann, G. (1973b). *British Journal of Anaesthesia*, **45**, 1097.

Doenicke, A., Wagner, E. and Beetz, K. H. (1973c). *Anaesthesist*, **22**, 353.

Duhm, B., Maul, W., Medenwald, H., Patzschke, K. and Wegner, L. A. (1965). *Anaesthesiologie und Wiederbelebung*, **4**, 78.

Dundee, J. W. (1960). *British Journal of Anaesthesia*, **32**, 407.

Dundee, J. W. (1963). *British Journal of Anaesthesia*, **35**, 786.

Dundee, J. W. (1965a). *In* "General Anaesthesia" (Eds F. T. Evans and T. C. Gray), vol. 1, p. 493. Butterworths, London.

Dundee, J. W. (1965b). *In* "General Anaesthesia" (Eds F. T. Evans and T. C. Gray), vol. 1, p. 507. Butterworths, London.

Dundee, J. W. (1971). *Anesthesiology*, **35**, 137.

Dundee, J. W. and Clarke, R. S. J. (1964). *British Journal of Anaesthesia*, **36**, 100.

Dundee, J. W. and Clarke, R. S. J. (1973). *Lancet*, **i**, 831.

Dundee, J. W. and Wyant, G. M. (1974). "Intravenous Anaesthesia". Churchill Livingstone, Edinburgh and London.

Dundee, J. W., Bovill, J., Knox, J. W. D., Clarke, R. S. J., Black, G. W., Love, S. H. S., Moore, J., Elliott, J., Pandit, S. K. and Coppel, D. L. (1970). *Lancet*, **i**, 1370.

Dundee, J. W., Assem, E. S. K., Gaston, J. M., Keilty, S. R., Sutton, J. A., Clarke, R. S. J. and Grainger, D. (1974). *British Medical Journal*, **i**, 63.

Evans, J. M., Aspinall, K. W. and Hendy, P. G. (1972). *Journal of Small Animal Practice*, **13**, 479.

Eyring, H., Woodbury, J. W. and D'Arrigo, J. S. (1973). *Anesthesiology*, **38**, 415.

Figdor, S. K., Kodet, M. J., Bloom, B. M., Agnello, E. J., P'an, S. Y. and Laubach, G. D. (1957). *Journal of Pharmacology and Experimental Therapeutics*, **119**, 299.

Foley, E. I., Walton, B., Savege, T. M., Strunin, L. and Simpson, B. R. (1972). *Postgraduate Medical Journal*, **48**, Supplement (2), 112.

Fordham, R. M. M., Awdry, P. N. and Paterson, G. M. (1972). *Postgraduate Medical Journal*, **48**, Supplement (2), 129.

Frey, R. (1971). *Anaesthesist*, **20**, 487.

Galley, A. H. and Lerman, L. H. (1959). *British Medical Journal*, **i**, 332.

Galley, A. H. and Rooms, M. (1956). *Lancet*, **i**, 990.

Gibbs, J. M. (1972). *British Journal of Anaesthesia*, **44**, 1298.

Gibson, W. R., Swanson, E. E. and Doran, W. J. (1955). *Proceedings of the Society for Experimental Biology and Medicine*, **89**, 292.

Gibson, W. R., Doran, W. J., Wood, W. C. and Swanson, E. E. (1959). *Journal of Pharmacology and Experimental Therapeutics*, **125**, 23.

Gilbert, H. G., Woollett, E. A. and Child, K. J. (1973). *Journal of Reproduction and Fertility*, **34**, 519.

Glen, J. B. (1973). *Veterinary Record*, **92**, 65.

Glickman, P. B., Palmer, R. H. and Kappas, A. (1964). *Archives of Internal Medicine*, **114**, 46.

Gordan, G. S., Guardagni, N., Picchi, J. and Adams, J. E. (1955). *Médecine et Hygiène (Genève)*, No. 297, 251.

Gordh, T. (1971). *Anaesthesist*, **20**, 481.

Gram, T. E. and Gillette, J. R. (1971). *In* "Fundamentals of Biochemical Pharmacology" (Ed. Z. M. Bacq), p. 571. Pergamon Press, Oxford.

Gruber, C. M., Stoelting, V. K., Forney, R. B., White, P. and De Meyer, M. (1957). *Anesthesiology*, **18**, 50.

Gyermek, L. (1967). *Proceedings of the Society for Experimental Biology and Medicine*, **125**, 1058.

Gyermek, L., Iriarte, J. and Crabbé, P. (1968). *Journal of Medicinal Chemistry*, **11**, 117.

Hall, L. W. C. (1972). *Postgraduate Medical Journal*, **48**, Supplement (2), 55.

Hall, L. W., Trim, C. M. and Woolf, N. (1972). *British Medical Journal*, **ii**, 145.

Halsey, M. J. and Kent, D. W. (1972). *Anesthesiology*, **36**, 313.

Halsey, M. J., Millar, R. A. and Sutton, J. A. (1974). "Molecular Mechanisms in General Anaesthesia". Churchill Livingstone, Edinburgh, London and New York.

Harrison, G. G. (1973). *British Journal of Anaesthesia*, **45**, 1019.

Henschel, W. F. and Buhr, G. (1965). *Anaesthesiologie und Wiederbelebung*, **4**, 227.

Hester, J. B. (1973). *British Journal of Anaesthesia*, **45**, 303.

Hewitt, J. C., Hamilton, R. C., O'Donnell, J. F. and Dundee, J. W. (1966). *British Journal of Anaesthesia*, **38**, 115.

Hidalgo, J., Dileo, R. M., Rikimaru, M. T., Guzman, R. J. and Thompson, C. R. (1971). *Anesthesia and Analgesia (Cleveland), Current Researches*, **50**, 231.

Hiltmann, R., Wollweber, H., Wirth, W. and Hoffmeister, F. (1965). *Anaesthesiologie und Wiederbelebung*, **4**, 1.

Hoffmeister, F., Grünvogel, E. and Wirth, W. (1965). *Anaesthesiologie und Wiederbelebung*, **4**, 88.

Horton, J. N. (1973). *Anaesthesia*, **28**, 182.

Howells, T. H., Odell, J. R., Hawkins, T. J. and Steane, P. A. (1964). *British Journal of Anaesthesia*, **36**, 295.

Howells, T. H., Harnik, E., Kellner, G. A. and Rosenoer, V. M. (1967). *British Journal of Anaesthesia*, **39**, 31.

Isaacs, H. and Barlow, M. B. (1973). *British Journal of Anaesthesia*, **45**, 901.

Jailer, J. W. and Goldbaum, L. R. (1946). *Journal of Laboratory and Clinical Medicine*, **31**, 1344.

Janssen, P. A. J., Niemegeers, C. J. E., Schellekens, K. H. L. and Lenaerts, F. M. (1971). *Arzneimittel-Forschung*, **21**, 1234.

Jarvis, C. A. N. (1972). *British Journal of Anaesthesia*, **44**, 989.

Johnstone, M. and Barron, P. T. (1968). *Anaesthesia*, **23**, 180.

Johnstone, M., Evans, V. and Baigel, S. (1959). *British Journal of Anaesthesia*, **31**, 433.

Kappas, A. and Palmer, R. H. (1963). *Pharmacological Reviews*, **15**, 123.

Kappas, A. and Palmer, R. H. (1965). *In* "Methods in Hormone Research" (Ed. R. I. Dorfman), vol. 4, p. 1. Academic Press, New York and London.

Kappas, A., Hellman, L., Fukushima, D. K. and Gallagher, T. F. (1957). *Journal of Clinical Endocrinology and Metabolism*, **17**, 451.

Kappas, A., Soybel, W., Fukushima, D. K. and Gallagher, T. F. (1959). *Transactions of the Association of American Physicians*, **72**, 54.

Kappas, A., Soybel, W., Glickman, P. and Fukushima, D. K. (1960). *Archives of Internal Medicine*, **105**, 701.

Krantz, J. C., Carr, C. J., Bird, J. G. and Cook, S. (1948). *Journal of Pharmacology and Experimental Therapeutics*, **93**, 188.

Krantz, J. C., Carr, C. J., Bubert, H. M. and Bird, J. G. (1949). *Journal of Pharmacology and Experimental Therapeutics*, **97**, 125.

Kroll, W. (1962). *International Zoo Yearbook*, **4**, 131.

Kruger, H. W. (1970). *Geburtschilfe und Frauenheilkunde*, **30**, 37.

Kurz, H. (1966). *Naunyn-Schmiedebergs Archiv fuer Experimentelle Pathologie und Pharmakologie*, **255**, 33.

Laborit, H., Huguenard, P., Douzon, C., Weber, B. and Guittard, R. (1956). *Archives Internationales de Pharmacodynamie et de Thérapie*, **107**, 159.

Laborit, H., Jouany, J., Gerard, J. and Fabiani, F. (1960). *La Presse Medicale*, **68**, 1867.

Langrehr, D. (1965). *Anaesthesiologie und Wiederbelebung*, **4**, 239.

Laubach, G. D., P'an, S. Y. and Rudel, H. W. (1955). *Science*, **122**, 78.

Lerman, L. H. and Paton, W. D. M. (1960). *British Journal of Pharmacology*, **15**, 458.

Liebegott, G. (1965). *Anaesthesiologie und Wiederbelebung*, **4**, 125.

List, W. F., Crumrine, R. S., Cascorbi, H. F. and Weiss, M. H. (1972). *Anesthesiology*, **36**, 98.

Lorenz, W., Doenicke, A., Meyer, R., Reimann, H. J., Kusche, J., Barth, H., Geesing, H., Hutzel, M. and Weissenbacher, B. (1972). *British Journal of Anaesthesia*, **44**, 355.

Lundy, J. S. (1935). *Proceedings of the Staff Meetings of the Mayo Clinic*, **10**, 536.

Mark, L. C. (1963). *Clinical Pharmacology and Therapeutics*, **4**, 504.

Mark, L. C., Burns, J. J., Brand, L., Campomanes, C. I., Trousof, N., Papper, E. M. and Brodie, B. B. (1958). *Journal of Pharmacology and Experimental Therapeutics*, **123**, 70.

Mark, L. C., Brand, L., Kamvyssi, S., Britton, R. C., Perel, J. M., Landrau, M. A. and Dayton, P. G. (1965). *Nature*, **206**, 1117.

Mark, L. C., Perel, J. M., Brand, L. and Dayton, P. G. (1968). *Anesthesiology*, **29**, 1159.

Mark, L. C., Perel, J. M., Brand, L. and Dayton, P. G. (1969). *Anesthesiology*, **31**, 384.

Mark, L. C., Perel, J. M. and Brand, L. (1972). *Anesthesiology*, **36**, 412.

McCarthy, D. A., Chen, G., Kaump, D. H. and Ensor, C. (1965). *Journal of New Drugs*, **5**, 21.

Mehta, S. (1973). *Anaesthesia*, **28**, 669.

Merryman, W., Boiman, R., Barnes, L. and Rothchild, I. (1954). *Journal of Clinical Endocrinology and Metabolism*, **14**, 1567.

Miller, D. C., Bradford, E. M. W. and Campbell, D. (1972a). *Postgraduate Medical Journal*, **48**, Supplement (2), 133.

Miller, K. W., Paton, W. D. M. and Smith, E. B. (1965). *Nature*, **206**, 574.

Miller, K. W., Paton, W. D. M., Smith, E. B. and Smith, R. A. (1972b). *Anesthesiology*, **36**, 339.

Monks, P. S. and Norman, J. (1972). *British Journal of Anaesthesia*, **44**, 1303.

Morgan, M., Loh, L., Singer, L. and Moore, P. H. (1971). *Anaesthesia*, **26**, 158.

Mullins, L. J. (1973). *Anesthesiology*, **38**, 205.

Murphy, F. J., Guardagny, N. P. and Debon, F. (1955a). *Médecine et Hygiène (Genève)*, No. 297, 252.

Murphy, F. J., Guadagni, N. P. and DeBon, F. (1955b). *Journal of the American Medical Association*, **158**, 1412.

Nishimura, N. (1962). *Anesthesia and Analgesia (Cleveland), Current Researches*, **41**, 265.

Notcutt, W. G. (1973). *Anaesthesia*, **28**, 673.

P'an, S. Y. and Laubach, G. D. (1964). *In* "Methods in Hormone Research" (Ed. R. I. Dorfman), vol. 3, p. 415. Academic Press, New York and London.

P'an, S. Y., Gardocki, J. F., Hutcheon, D. E., Rudel, H., Kodet, M. J. and Laubach, G. D. (1955). *Journal of Pharmacology and Experimental Therapeutics*, **115**, 432.

Paton, W. D. M. and Payne, J. P. (1968). *In* "Pharmacological Principles and Practice", p. 71. Churchill, London.

Payne, J. P. and Wright, D. A. (1962). *British Journal of Anaesthesia*, **34**, 368.

Pickerodt, V. W. A., McDowall, D. G., Coroneos, N. J. and Keaney, N. P. (1972). *British Journal of Anaesthesia*, **44**, 751.

Price, H. L. (1960). *Anesthesiology*, **21**, 40.

Price, H. L., Dundee, J. W. and Conner, E. H. (1957). *Anesthesiology*, **18**, 171.

Price, H. L., Kovnak, P. H., Safer, J. N., Conner, E. H. and Price, M. L. (1960). *Clinical Pharmacology and Therapeutics*, **1**, 16.

Primo, J. and Lahon, H. (1965). *Anesthesia Analgesie Réanimation*, **22**, 417.

Pütter, J. (1965). *Anaesthesiologie und Wiederbelebung*, **4**, 61.

Reid, J. S. and Frank, R. J. (1972). *Journal of American Animal Hospitals Association*, **8**, 115.

Riding, J. E., Dundee, J. W., Rajagopalan, M. S., Hamilton, R. C. and Baskett, P. J. F. (1963). *British Journal of Anaesthesia*, **35**, 480.

Robertson, J. D. and Wynn Williams, A. (1961). *Anaesthesia*, **16**, 389.

Rozenkranz, I. (1972). *British Journal of Anaesthesia*, **44**, 1332.

Saidman, L. J. and Eger, E. I. (1966). *Anesthesiology*, **27**, 118.

Savege, T. M., Foley, E. I., Coultas, R. J., Walton, B., Strunin, L., Simpson, R. B. and Scott, D. F. (1971). *Anaesthesia*, **26**, 402.

Selye, H. (1941a). *Proceedings of the Society for Experimental Biology and Medicine*, **46**, 116.

Selye, H. (1941b). *Journal of Pharmacology and Experimental Therapeutics*, **73**, 127.

Selye, H. (1942). *Endocrinology*, **30**, 437.

Shapiro, H. M., Wyte, S. R. and Harris, A. B. (1972). *British Journal of Anaesthesia*, **44**, 1200.

Shideman, F. E., Gould, T. C., Winters, W. D., Peterson, R. C. and Wilner, W. K. (1953). *Journal of Pharmacology and Experimental Therapeutics*, **107**, 368.

Stoelting, V. K. (1957). *Anesthesia and Analgesia (Cleveland), Current Researches*, **36**, 49.

Swerdlow, M. (1961). *British Journal of Anaesthesia*, **33**, 104.

Swerdlow, M. (1962). *British Journal of Anaesthesia*, **34**, 558.

Swerdlow, M., Chakraborty, S. K. and Zahangir, M. A. H. M. (1971). *British Journal of Anaesthesia*, **43**, 1075.

Szappanyos, G. G., Bopp, P. and Fournet, P. C. (1969). *Anaesthesist*, **18**, 365.

Takahashi, T., Takasaki, M., Namiki, A. and Dohi, S. (1973). *British Journal of Anaesthesia*, **45**, 179.

Takki, S., Nikki, P., Jäättelä, A. and Tammisto, T. (1972). *British Journal of Anaesthesia*, **44**, 1318.

Taylor, C. and Stoelting, V. K. (1960). *Anesthesiology*, **21**, 29.

Taylor, P. A., Towey, R. M. and Rappoport, A. S. (1972). *British Journal of Anaesthesia*, **44**, 1163.

Thuillier, M. J. and Domenjoz, R. (1957). *Anaesthesist*, **6**, 163.

Thurmon, J. C., Nelson, D. R. and Christie, G. J. (1972). *Journal American Veterinary Medical Association*, **160**, 1325.
Torda, T. A., Burkhart, J. and Toh, W. (1972). *Anaesthesia*, **27**, 159.
Traber, D. L., Priano, L. L. and Wilson, R. S. (1970). *Journal of Pharmacology and Experimental Therapeutics*, **175**, 395.
Turner, K. J., Keep, V. R. and Bartholomaeus, N. (1972). *British Journal of Anaesthesia*, **44**, 211.
Turner, J. M., Coroneos, N. J., Gibson, R. M., Powell, D., Ness, M. A. and McDowall, D. G. (1973). *British Journal of Anaesthesia*, **45**, 168.
Tweed, W. A., Minuck, M. and Mymin, D. (1972). *Anesthesiology*, **37**, 613.
Vickers, M. D. (1969). *International Anesthesiology Clinics*, **7**, 75.
Virtue, R. W., Alanis, J. M., Mori, M., Lafargue, R. T., Vogel, J. H. K. and Metcalf, D. R. (1967). *Anesthesiology*, **28**, 823.
Walker, A. K. Y. (1972). *Anaesthesia*, **27**, 408.
Warren, J. B. (1972). *Postgraduate Medical Journal*, **48**, Supplement (2), 130.
Waters, D. J. (1966). *Anaesthesia*, **21**, 346.
Weis, K. H. and Ruckes, J. (1965). *Anaesthesiologie und Wiederbelebung*, **4**, 108.
Weston Hurst, E. (1958). *In* "A Symposium on the Evaluation of Drug Toxicity" (Eds. A. L. Walpole and A. Spinks), p. 12. Churchill, London.
Wilson, R. D., Traber, D. L., Barrett, E., Creson, D. L., Schmitt, R. C. and Allen, C. R. (1970). *Anesthesia and Analgesia (Cleveland), Current Researches*, **49**, 236.
Wirth, W. and Hoffmeister, F. (1965). *Anaesthesiologie und Wiederbelebung*, **4**, 17.
Witzel, H. (1959). *Zeitschrift fuer Vitamin, Hormon und Fermentforschung*, **10**, 46.
Wright, D. A. and Payne, J. P. (1962). *British Journal of Anaesthesia*, **34**, 379.
Wyte, S. R., Shaprio, H. M., Turner, P. and Harris, A. B. (1972). *Anesthesiology*, **36**, 174.

Steroidal Neuromuscular Blocking Agents

W. R. BUCKETT, BPharm, PhD, FPS[1]

*Pharmacology Section, Imperial Chemical Industries Ltd,
Pharmaceuticals Division, Alderley Park,
Cheshire, England*

1   Introduction

As with so many areas of drug research, new approaches to rational drug design have arisen from a consideration of natural product chemistry and pharmacology. The development and use of steroidal neuromuscular blocking agents indeed commenced in this fashion with natural products such as conessine (3β-dimethylaminocon-5-ene) being isolated and quaternary derivatives being prepared even in the last century (Polstorff and Schirmer, 1886). However it was the pharmacological evaluation of conessine and close analogues (Burn, 1914; Stephenson, 1948) which led to a greater interest in this type of compound for producing neuromuscular blockade.

---

[1] Present address: Novo A/S, 2880-Bagsvaerd, Copenhagen, Denmark.

Several years later a resurgence of interest in the area was brought about by the isolation and pharmacological evaluation of the steroidal alkaloid malouétine (Janot *et al.*, 1960) which is a naturally occurring bisquaternary ammonium salt. At about this time synthetic efforts around the androstane nucleus led to dipyrandium chloride ($3\beta,17\beta$-dipyrrolidin-1'-yl-5α-androstane dimethochloride) which was expected to be of short duration (Biggs *et al.*, 1964). Similar synthetic work on conessine yielded the putative short-acting drug, *NN'*-dimethylconessine from a large series (Busfield *et al.*, 1968).

A more rational approach to neuromuscular blocking drugs involved the incorporation of a fragment from the naturally occurring neurotransmitter acetylcholine into naturally occurring androstane compounds (Hewett and Savage, 1968) to yield curarizing drugs, although of low potency. Incorporation of two acetylcholine fragments according to classical concepts led to compounds of great interest from the point of view of potency and specificity of action (Buckett *et al.*, 1967). One of these compounds, pancuronium bromide (Buckett *et al.*, 1968), was considered to be of value in anaesthesia and is now clinically accepted as a standard drug (Speight and Avery, 1972).

It is with the development of these various classes of neuromuscular blocking drugs, their chemistry and pharmacology that this review is principally concerned. It is the first time that a review has been compiled on the subject of steroidal neuromuscular blocking agents.

2 Naturally occurring steroidal alkaloids and their derivatives

2.1 MALOUÉTINE AND ITS DERIVATIVES

In 1960 Janot *et al.* isolated two steroidal alkaloids from *Malouetia berquaertiana* (Apocynaceae), funtuphyllamine B and malouétine. Funtuphyllamine B ($20S$)-3β-hydroxymethylamino-5α-pregnane (1)[1] is a weak secondary base common to several tropical species and lacking any

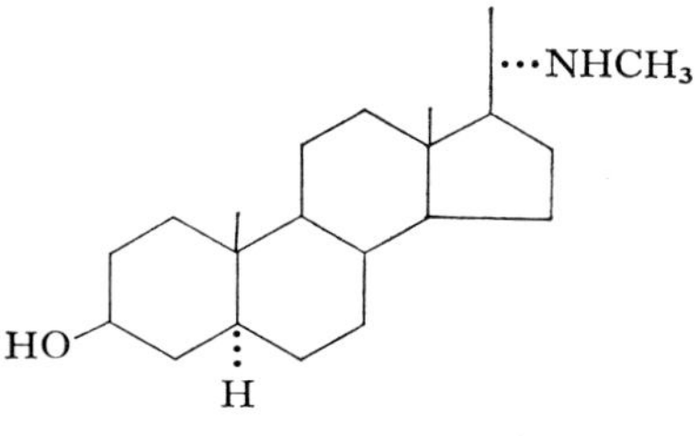

(1) 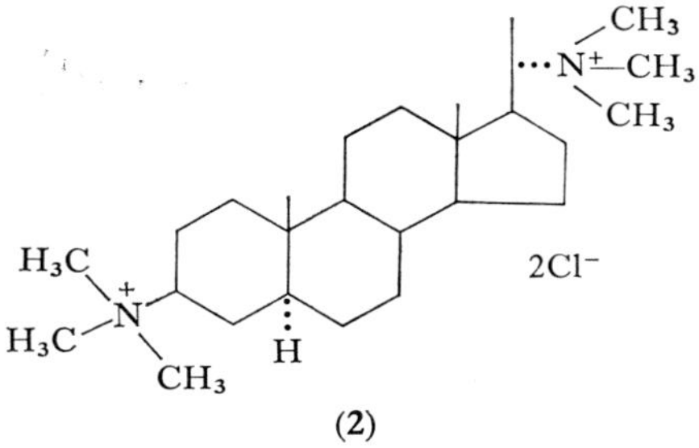   (2)

[1] The configuration at position **20** is depicted as a Fischer projection, but with the highest numbered carbon at the top.

marked pharmacological action. Malouétine (20S)-3β-bistrimethylamino-5α-pregnane dimethochloride (2) is the compound which is responsible for the pronounced curarizing action seen with the plant extract.

The pharmacology of malouétine was first studied by Quevauviller and Lainé (1960) who showed it to be one-third as toxic as tubocurarine intravenously in mice, while being of similar potency in producing neuromuscular blockade in the cat sciatic nerve-tibialis muscle preparation. Thus malouétine has a more favourable ratio of activity to toxicity than tubocurarine and in efforts to improve this still further the stereoisomers of malouétine were resolved (Janot et al., 1962) and subjected to a comparative pharmacological study. Khuong-Huu et al. (1964) using the conscious rabbit head-drop test showed that 3β-trimethylamino substitution was preferable to 3α-substitution for potency, whereas the 3α-isomers had a slightly shorter duration of action (Table 1). Further work on the duration of neuromuscular blockade due to malouétine suggested that the drug would be of intermediate duration between that of gallamine and

TABLE 1

The potency and duration of action of malouétine, its stereoisomers and other neuromuscular blocking agents in the rabbit

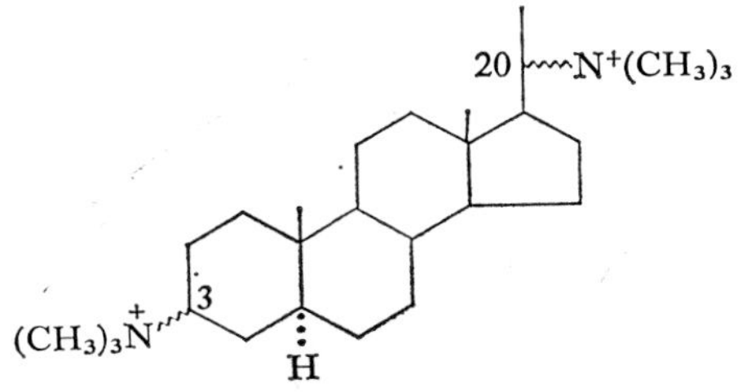

Compound	Configuration of substituents 3	20	Neuromuscular blocking dose[a] mg kg^{-1}	Lethal dose[a] mg kg^{-1}	Duration of 10 times lethal dose[b] min
Malouétine	β	S	0·15	0·20	25
	β	R	0·15	0·20	25
	α	S	0·20	0·30	20
	α	R	0·20	0·30	21
Tubocurarine			0·18	0·20	120
Gallamine			0·40	0·60	105
Suxamethonium			0·30	0·50	20

[a] Conscious animals.
[b] Anaesthetized animals.

suxamethonium. It is of nondepolarizing mode of action since reversal is effected by neostigmine and muscle contracture is absent in avians. No cumulative action was apparent in the dog in which species 0·5 mg kg⁻¹ gave 100 per cent blockade of the neuromuscular junction. At this dose marked hypotension was evident and at 1 mg kg⁻¹ pronounced EKG changes (flattened QRS wave) and bradycardia, which were irreversible after 5 mg kg⁻¹, were observed. Malouétine and its stereoisomers were not therefore studied clinically.

Monoquaternary methylsulphate derivatives of the related alkaloids funtumine (3) and funtumidine (4) have been prepared and examined in cats and rabbits (Blanpin and Bretaudeau, 1961). They were 1/55th and 1/75th as potent as tubocurarine respectively and did not evoke much interest.

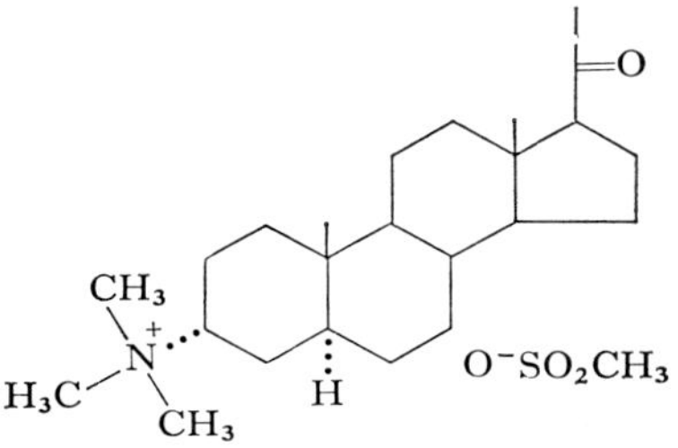

(3) 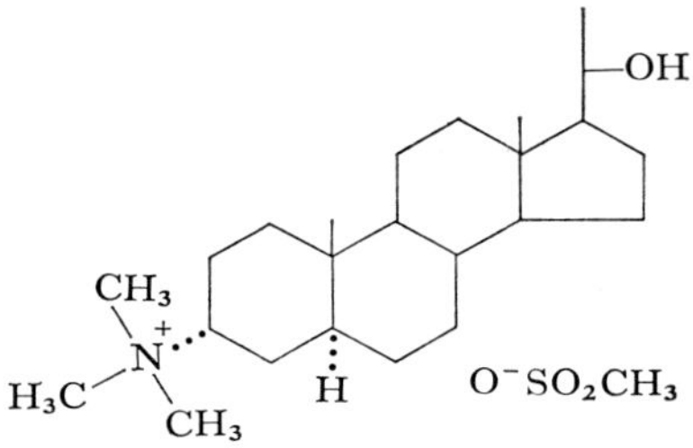   (4)

2.2   CONESSINE AND PARAVALLARIDINE DERIVATIVES

Although the pharmacological properties of conessine (3β-dimethyl-aminocon-5-ene) (5) and its isomers were described, neuromuscular blockade demonstrated (Stephenson, 1948) and quaternary salts prepared (Polstorff and Schirmer, 1886; Bertho, 1944), no extensive pharmacological evaluation of conessine analogues was carried out until the work of

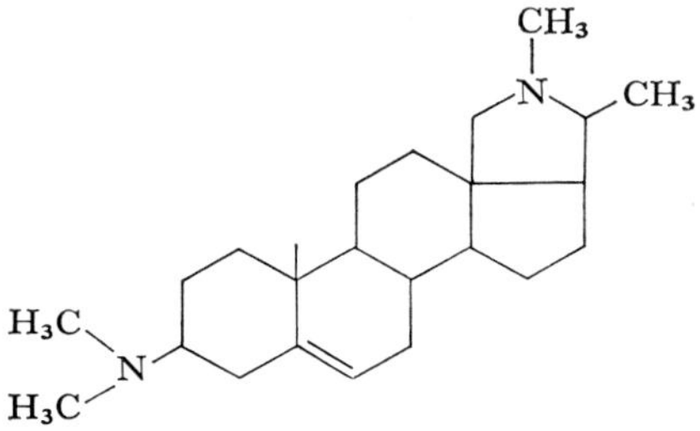

(5) 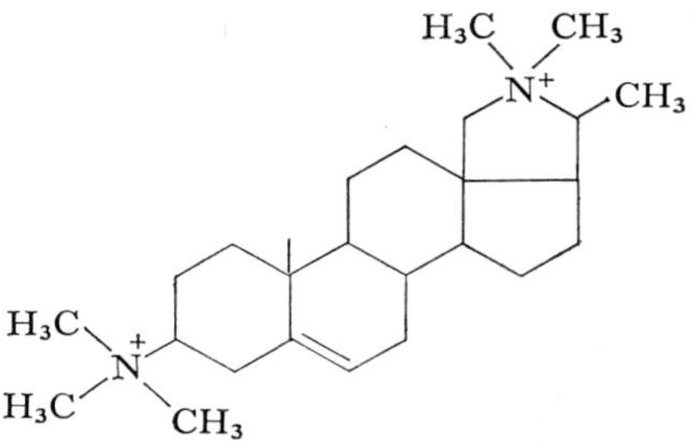   (6)

Busfield *et al.* (1968). Twenty-six derivatives of conessine, both mono-quaternary and bisquaternary salts, were examined and NN'-dimethyl-conessine (**6**) was described in detail.

Reference to the selected compounds listed in Table 2 will give an indication of the range of neuromuscular blocking potency obtained. Whereas an increase in alkylation on the quaternary nitrogen of the mono-quaternary derivatives increased potency, this progression was not observed

TABLE 2

Neuromuscular blocking activity of conessine derivatives assessed on the anaesthetized cat tibialis preparation

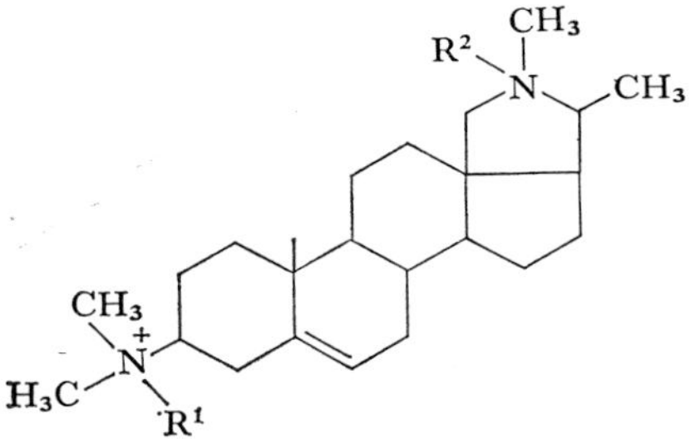

NN' substitution		Relative potency
R_1	R_2	(tubocurarine $= 1\cdot0$)
CH_3	—	0·12
C_2H_5	—	0·33
C_4H_9	—	0·64
CH_2Ph	—	0·58
CH_2CH_2OPh	—	0·45
O	—	0·02
CH_3	CH_3	0·62
C_2H_5	C_2H_5	0·79
C_3H_7	C_3H_7	0·47
CH_2Ph	CH_2Ph	0·51
$CH(CH_3)_2$	CH_3	1·61
C_4H_9	CH_3	1·54
CH_2Ph	CH_3	1·09
CH_2CH_2OPh	CH_3	1·37

with the bisquaternary compounds, most of which were approximately half as potent as tubocurarine. If, however, the N' position was quatern-ized by a methyl group, larger groupings at 3α yielded compounds of greater potency than tubocurarine. All the compounds examined had a reasonable short duration of action, though generally longer than that of malouétine.

The pharmacology of *NN'*-dimethylconessine (6) was of considerable interest in that these authors found the compound to be of comparable potency to tubocurarine and with a qualitatively similar mode of action, yet to have a short duration of action equivalent to that of suxamethonium in the cat. In the monkey there appeared to be a somewhat slower recovery rate than in the cat and this was subsequently borne out in clinical studies (Verner, 1963). Although of rapid onset, the action of *NN'*-dimethylconessine was of three times the duration of suxamethonium, so clinical studies were abandoned even though adverse cardiovascular effects were absent.

(7)

The monoquaternary compound cona-3,5-dienine ethiodide or stercuronium (7) was first reported by Wieriks (1969) to be a nondepolarizing neuromuscular blocker with duration of action lying between that of suxamethonium and gallamine in cats and monkeys. After intravenous injection in guinea pigs bronchoconstriction was absent suggesting lack of histamine-releasing properties. Further analysis of the actions of stercuronium by Marshall (1973b) showed the onset of action to be more rapid than current clinically used blockers and that the ratio between the neuromuscular blocking dose and the ganglionic blocking dose was reasonably large (Marshall, 1973c). The cardiac vagolytic effect was not inconsiderable and has apparently precluded the use of this drug in anaesthesia. The short duration of this drug has been claimed to be due to its rapid uptake into liver and kidneys, with consequent fast decline in blood levels, as shown by whole body autoradiography in the rat (Hespe and Wieriks, 1971). It also appeared from this study that stercuronium is excreted unchanged in the rat, in which species it possesses only one-twelfth the potency of tubocurarine (Derkx *et al.*, 1971).

Compounds derived from the naturally occurring alkaloid paravallaridine (8), the second alkaloid of *Paravallaris microphylla* (Le Men *et al.*, 1963), have recently been prepared by a six-stage procedure from the natural

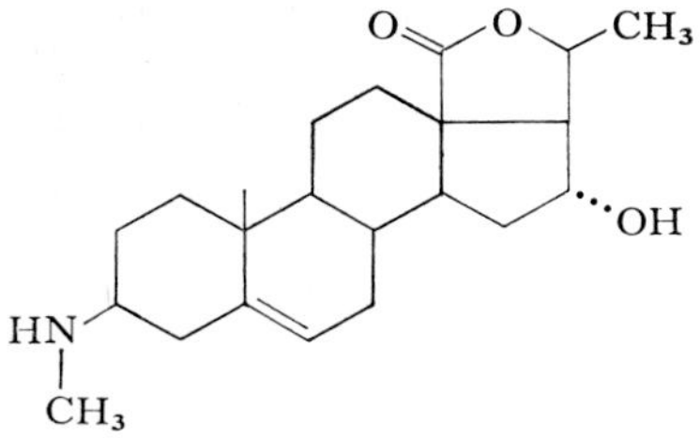

(8)

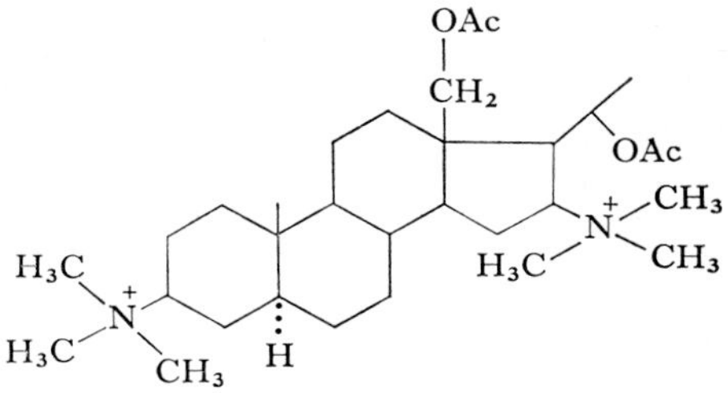

(9)

product, and Roquet *et al.* (1971) have reported on their activity. The stereoisomers (Table 3) show curarizing actions of the nondepolarizing type which are reversed by neostigmine. Optimal potency was secured with the bisquaternary (20*S*)-16β-diacetate (9), although the other configurations were almost as potent. If the 3β-nitrogen atom was tertiary then potency

TABLE 3

Biological activities of paravallaridine derivatives

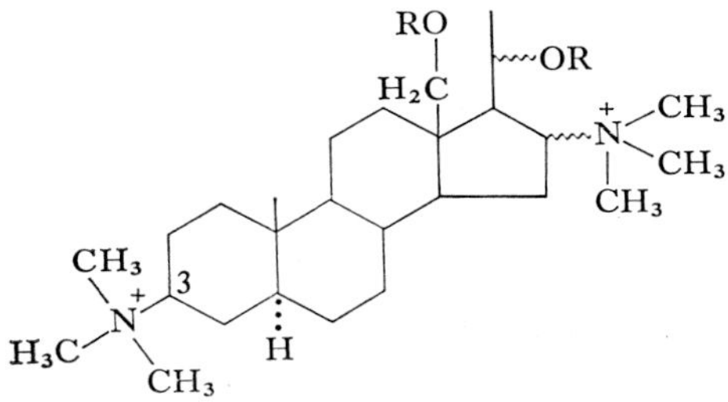

R	Configuration at 5	Configuration at 16	Configuration at 20	N valency at C-3	ED$_{50}$ mg kg^{-1} i.v. Cat tibialis	ED$_{50}$ mg kg^{-1} i.v. Rabbit head drop	LD$_{50}$ i.v. mg kg^{-1} mice
H	α	β	R	4	0·90	1·50	2·4
OAc	α	β	R	4	0·35	1·67	2·8
OAc	α	β	S	4	0·27	1·47	2·7
OAc	α	α	R	4	0·62	1·63	7·5
OAc	α	α	S	4	0·28	1·80	3·4
OAc	Δ^5	β	R	4	0·55	1·44	2·3
OAc	Δ^5	α	S	4	0·75	1·67	6·0
OAc	α	α	R	3	1·00	1·50	4·3
OAc	α	α	S	3	0·46	1·80	5·5

was reduced to half that of the equivalent bisquaternary compound; similar effects were found when the Δ^5-compounds were compared with the saturated 5α-compounds. Finally the absence of acetylation at 18 and

20 reduced the potency. However, all the paravallaridine derivatives lie within a narrow four-fold range of potency similar to tubocurarine unlike most other series considered in this chapter, in which the spread of potency is very much greater.

3   Drugs based on the androstane nucleus

3.1   DIPYRANDIUM, ITS STEREOISOMERS AND ANALOGUES

The pharmacological report of Biggs *et al.* (1964) suggested that dipyrandium chloride (3β,17β-dipyrrolid-1'-yl-5α-androstane dimethochloride) (M & B 9105A) (10) would be of interest due to the short duration and non-depolarizing mode of action exhibited in several species such as rabbit,

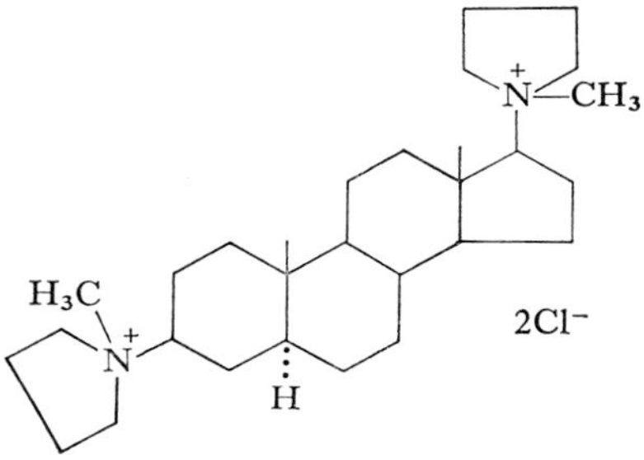

(10)

cat and hen, while being of similar potency to tubocurarine. It was therefore given a clinical investigation by Mushin and Mapleson (1964).

However in man, when the drug was tested in conscious volunteers by stimulating the median nerve at the wrist and recording the near-isometric tension developed by the short muscles of the thumb, recovery from the neuromuscular blocking action was very variable and never as rapid as the recovery following the depolarizing drug suxamethonium. In addition a fairly consistent rise in heart rate was observed. The findings agreed with the pharmacological prediction from monkeys and suggest that this may be the species of choice when assessing duration of action of these drugs.

The use of this type of quaternary aminoandrostane to deduce some characteristics of the possible receptor for neuromuscular blocking agents has been attempted by two groups of workers (Alauddin *et al.*, 1965; Bamford *et al.*, 1967, 1971) since the steroidal skeleton can afford a reasonably rigid backbone for support of the ammonium functions. Alauddin *et al.* (1965) studied substitution of the quaternary ammonium heads at the 3α and 17α-positions of diamino-5α- androstane derivatives (**11**). A four or five carbon substitution (**11**b and **11**c) appears optimal for activity,

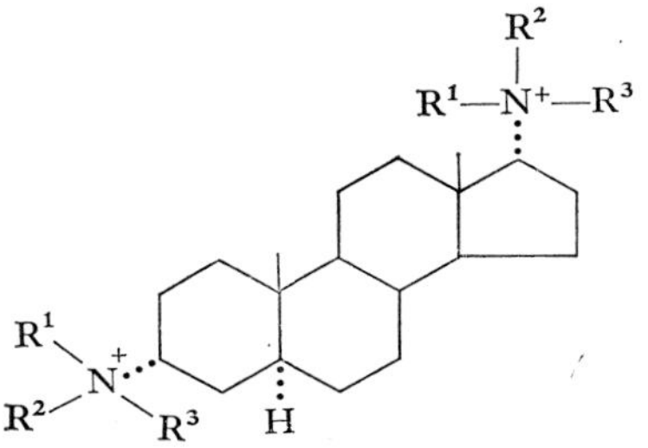

(**11**)

suggesting that charge density and also lipophilicity are important (Table 4). Other studies (Martin-Smith, 1971) showed that the potency varied little when β-substitution at 3 and 17 was effected. In extending this approach stereoisomerically Bamford *et al.* (1967) studied the eight isomers

TABLE 4

The neuromuscular blocking potency of $3\alpha,17\alpha$-diamino-5α-androstane derivatives (**11**) in the cat

Compound (11)	R_1	R_2	R_3	Molar blocking potency[a] (tubocurarine = 1·0)
a	CH_3	CH_3	CH_3	0·27
b	CH_3	C_2H_5	CH_3	0·84
c	C_2H_5	C_2H_5	CH_3	0·87
d	C_2H_5	C_2H_5	C_2H_5	0·46

[a] Cat sciatic-gastrocnemius preparation.
From Alauddin *et al.* (1965).

of dipyrandium (**10**) derived by varying positions 3, 5 and 17 (**12**). In these compounds the α-substitution of the steroid by the quaternary groupings should avoid steric hindrance of a possible drug–receptor interaction by the β-methyl groups at C-10 and C-13. However, α-substitution at all three positions (**12**d) led to a compound possessing only half the potency of the corresponding β-substituted derivative (**12**e) (Table 5). 3α-Substitution gave the least active compounds, whereas 17-substitution was less stereospecific in either the 5α or 5β-androstanes, so it is postulated that

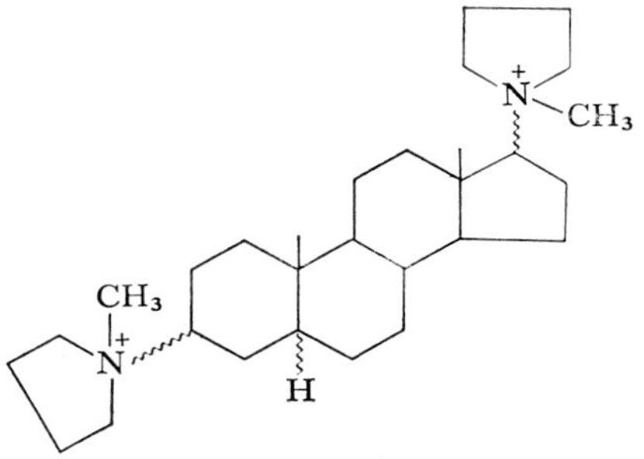

(12)

TABLE 5

Neuromuscular blocking potency of dipyrandium stereoisomers **(12)** in the cat

Compound (12)	Configuration of substituents			Molar blocking potency[a] (tubocurarine = 1·0)
	3	17	5	
a	β	β	α	0·76
b	β	α	α	0·76
c	α	β	α	0·43
d	α	α	α	0·33
e	β	β	β	0·67
f	β	α	β	0·51
g	α	β	β	0·07
h	α	α	β	0·07

[a] Cat sciatic-tibialis anterior preparation.
From Bamford et al. (1967).

the receptor interaction with the 3-position is more important than interaction in either 17-configuration. Corresponding monoquaternary androstanes have also been described by Bamford et al. (1971) and it was found that the 3-monoquaternary salts were generally more potent than 17-monoquaternary salts, again favouring the importance of the 3-position for determining potency.

3.2   2β,16β-DIAMINO-5α-ANDROSTANE DERIVATIVES

All the neuromuscular blocking agents described up to this point were the result of either isolation of natural products and semi-synthetic derivatives thereof or the result of using the steroidal nucleus purely as a supporting framework upon which to locate active centres such as the quaternary ammonium grouping. Buckett *et al.* (1967, 1973) have utilized the steroidal structure in a somewhat different way in the preparation of neuro-muscular blocking drugs. Their concept is of the incorporation of a naturally occurring biological neurotransmitter such as acetylcholine (13) in a rigid conformation directly into the steroidal skeleton in the hope that the well-tolerated resultant drug will perhaps penetrate to unique and specific sites of action in the body. This concept appears to be realized with pan-curonium bromide (*vide infra*).

The incorporation of acetylcholine fragments first commenced using 5α-androstan-17-one, incorporation of a single fragment taking place in ring-*A* (Hewett and Savage, 1968). The acetylcholine analogue (14) had only approximately one-seventieth the potency of tubocurarine in contrast to the cyclic piperidino analogue (15) which was one-sixteenth as potent (Lewis *et al.*, 1967). However, ganglionic blocking effects were also seen at the neuromuscular blocking dosage, so these compounds were taken purely as a starting point for further syntheses. In addition to the 2β-amino-5α-androstanes described above, four 3α-amino derivatives were also examined (Lewis *et al.*, 1967). Again the weak neuromuscular blocking actions coupled with ganglionic blockade were apparent, but the main point of interest emerging was that 3α-amino substitution was less favourable

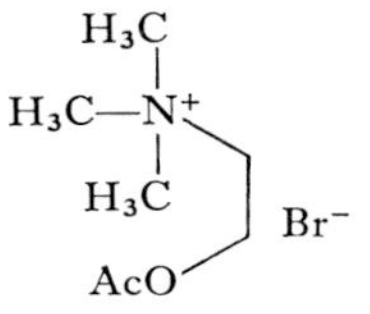

(13)

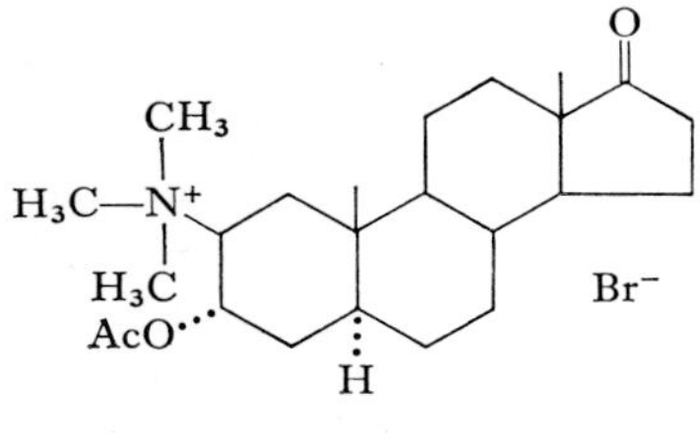

(14)

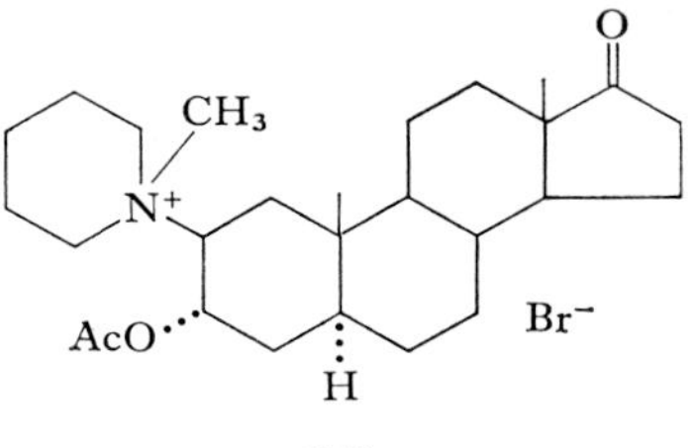

(15)

for potency than was 2β-amino substitution. This finding, together with the cyclic nitrogen requirement was borne in mind when bisamino compounds were later prepared. Compounds based on the pregnane skeleton, such as 3α-hydroxy-2β-piperidino-5α-pregnan-20-one methobromide, offered neither quantitative or qualitative advantages over the androstanes, probably because pregnanes are less hydrophilic.

The substitution of two acetylcholine fragments into the androstane nucleus gave rise to a very potent series of nondepolarizing neuromuscular blocking agents. Firstly, the influence of changing the substituent on the nitrogen was studied in the 3α,17β-diol derivatives (16). The dipiperidino

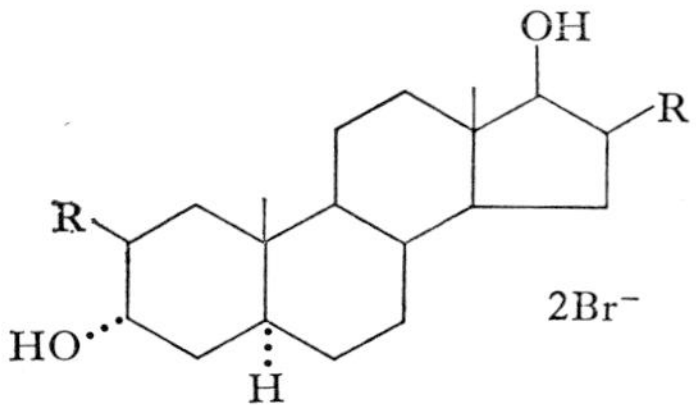

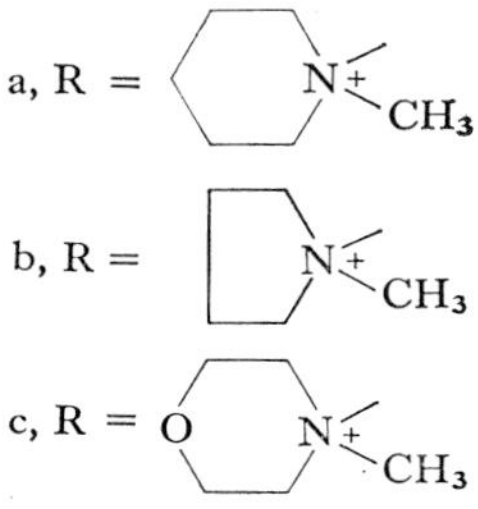

compound (16a) was half as potent and had half the duration of tubocurarine (in subsequent discussion in this section both potency and duration will always be discussed relative to tubocurarine and based on assessment in the anaesthetized cat sciatic-gastrocnemius preparation). Potency was reduced to 0·17 in the dipyrrolidino compound (16b) but the duration was also reduced to 0·32. The dimorpholino (16c) surprisingly was inactive, due perhaps to the charge dissipating effect of the oxygen atom in the morpholine ring.

The effects of various esterifications at the 3α,17β-diol positions were then examined (17 and Table 6). For high potency it is abundantly clear that esterification is indeed necessary, for both nonesterified derivatives (17a) and (17b) are less potent than tubocurarine. For potency esterification at 3 and 17 as diacetate (17g: pancuronium bromide) is optimal. Dipropionate (17j), dipivalate (17k), diformate (17d) and dibenzoate (17n) exhibit decreasing potency in that order probably due to increasing lipophilicity. The exception is the diformate which is probably rapidly hydrolysed to the diol (17a). As this diol has low potency and short duration in comparison with the diesters, it is possible that duration of action of the esters may depend on the hydrolysis rate of the 3- and 17-ester groupings: the dibenzoate is still active at 2 hours.

The 3-monoesters (17f, l, m) are generally shorter acting than the 17-monoester (17c) so it may be inferrred that the 3-esters hydrolyse more readily than 17-esters. This led to the development of dacuronium bromide (17f) for clinical trial and detailed investigation of Org-6368 (2β,16β-dipiperidino-5α-androstan-3α-ol acetate dimethobromide) (vide infra). It is also apparent from Table 6 that an ester grouping at 17 is a prerequisite

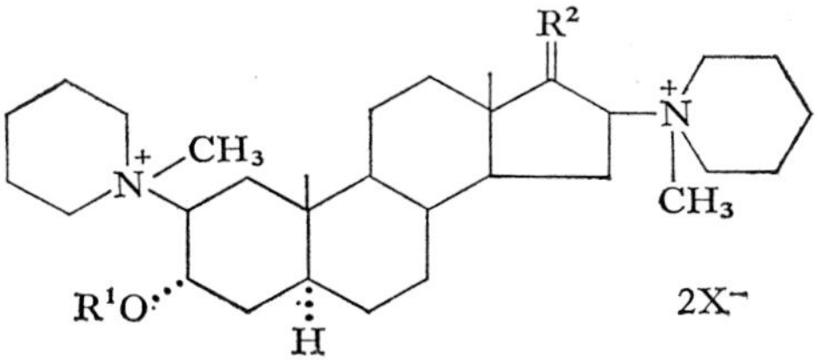

(17)

TABLE 6

Potency and duration of neuromuscular blocking action of $2\beta,16\beta$-dipiperidino-3,17-dioxy-5α-androstane dimethohalides (17)

Compound (17)	R_1	R_2	X	Neuromuscular blocking activity[a]	
				Potency	Duration
a	H	β-OH,H	Br	0·55	0·53
b	H	O	Br	0·67	0·47
c	H	β-CH$_3$COO,H	Br	5·15	1·00
d	CHO	β-CHO,H	Br	1·30	0·46
e	CH$_3$CO	O	Br	1·53	0·37
f	CH$_3$CO	β-OH,H	Br	1·72	0·49
g	CH$_3$CO	β-CH$_3$COO,H	Br	9·41	1·15
h	CH$_3$CO	β-C$_2$H$_5$COO,H	Br	5·60	0·85
i	CH$_3$CO	H,α-CH$_3$COO	Br	6·15	0·75
j	C$_2$H$_5$CO	β-C$_2$H$_5$COO,H	I	7·10	0·95
k	(CH$_3$)$_3$CCO	β-(CH$_3$)$_3$CCOO,H	I	3·80	1·47
l	(CH$_3$)$_3$CCO	β-OH,H	I	1·70	0·50
m	PhCO	β-OH,H	Br	0·84	0·72
n	PhCO	β-PhCOO,H	Br	1·00	3·00

[a] Relative potency (tubocurarine = 1·0) on cat sciatic-gastrocnemius preparation.
From Buckett et al. (1967, 1973).

for high potency, although this is generally associated with a longer duration of action.

Since the extremely long duration of toxiferine-C (**18**; R = CH$_3$) was shortened by diallyl quaternization to give alcuronium (**18**; R = CH$_2$CH=CH$_2$), similar unsaturated quaternization procedures were applied to the diacetate (**17g**) and diol (**17a**), but no significant shortening in duration of action was found.

Since the recent indication that although tubocurarine has a bisamino substitution, it is in fact a monoquaternary compound (Everett et al.,

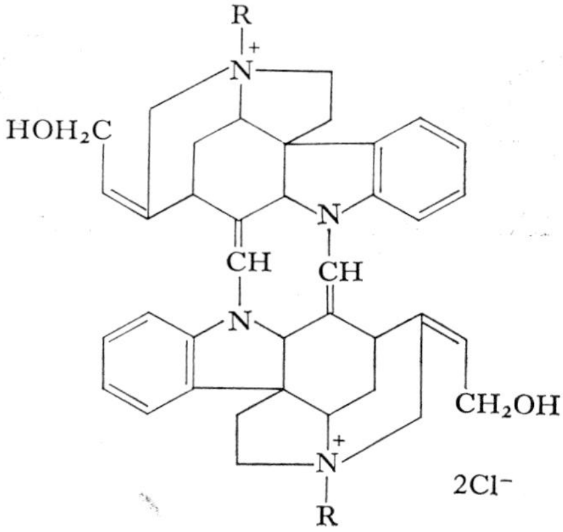

(18)

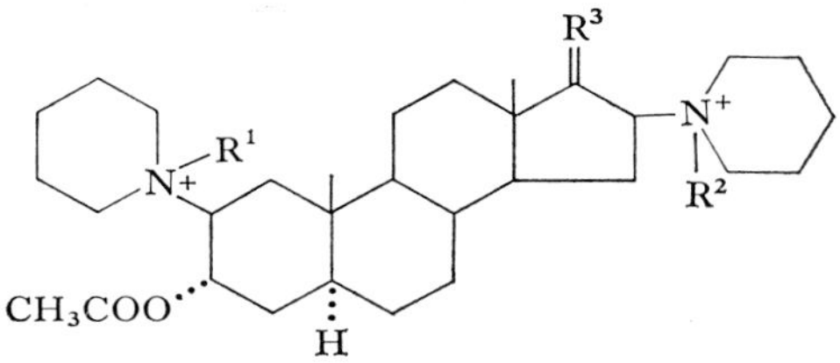

(19)

TABLE 7

Potency and duration of neuromuscular blocking action of $2\beta,16\beta$-dipiperidino-3,17-dioxy-5α-androstane di- and monomethobromides (19)

Compound (19)	R_1	R_2	R_3	Neuromuscular blocking activity[a] Potency	Duration
a	CH_3	CH_3	O	1·53	0·37
b	—	CH_3	O	0·39	0·44
c	CH_3	CH_3	β-OH,H	1·72	0·49
d	—	CH_3	β-OH,H	0·40	0·45
e	CH_3	CH_3	β-CH_3COO,H	9·41	1·15
f	—	CH_3	β-CH_3COO,H	6·00	0·77
g	CH_3	$CH_2CH{=}CH_2$	β-CH_3COO,H	7·23	1·16
h	—	$CH_2CH{=}CH_2$	β-CH_3COO,H	3·44	0·89

[a] Relative potency (tubocurarine = 1·0) on cat sciatic-gastrocnemius preparation.

1970) it was considered of interest by Buckett *et al.* (1967, 1973) to examine a few monoquaternary bisamino compounds (**19** and Table 7). In all cases the monoquaternary derivatives were less potent than the corresponding bisquaternaries, although some were much more potent than tubocurarine. Even in the absence of quaternization at position 3, sufficient ionization will take place at physiological pH to permit drug–receptor interaction to be effected and the blocking activity to be observed, albeit with somewhat reduced potency.

The most potent bisaminomonoquaternary compound (**19f**) was studied in some detail by Marshall (1968). In both the cat and the hen the potency was found to be about half that of the corresponding bisquaternary compound, pancuronium bromide (**19e**), and since the compound was about half the duration of action of tubocurarine it showed little or no cumulation and recovery following continuous intravenous infusion commenced immediately. In the rabbit, however, there was little difference in potency between mono- and bisquaternary compounds, in which species greater potency was seen than in the cat. The response to close-arterially injected acetylcholine was abolished in the cat tibialis anterior muscle. The blocking action was antagonized by neostigmine and was enhanced when the stimulation frequency was increased to one per second but no prolonged block of the hemicholinium type occurred. These results indicate that the block was solely postjunctional in origin and of a nondepolarizing nature.

3.3 DACURONIUM BROMIDE AND RELATED COMPOUNDS

3.3.1 *Introduction*

One of the objectives of the study outlined by Buckett *et al.* (1967; 1973) was the development of a steroidal neuromuscular blocking drug possessing a rapid onset and a short duration of action. In pharmacological studies dacuronium bromide (**20**) appeared to meet these requirements (Buckett and Saxena, 1969).

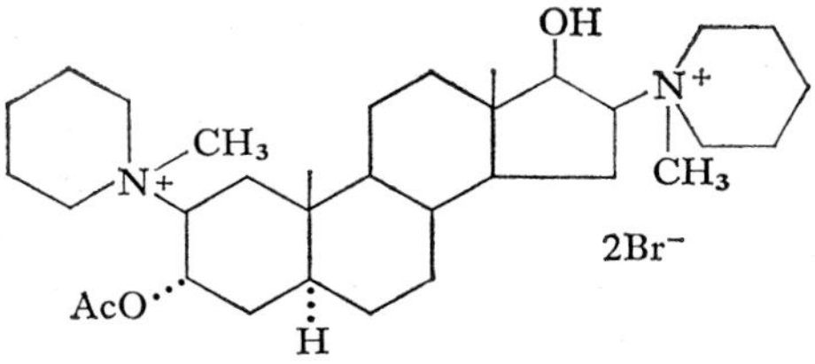

(**20**)

The compound is a short-acting neuromuscular blocker of nondepolarizing type having greater potency than tubocurarine in the cat, rabbit and dog, but not in the rat or the baboon (Table 8). Evidence for nondepolarizing

TABLE 8

The potency, onset and duration of action of dacuronium bromide (20) in the sciatic-gastrocnemius preparation of various anaesthetized animal species

Species	Effective neuro-muscular blocking dose mg kg^{-1}	Potency ± s.d.	Onset ± s.d. (tubocurarine = 1·0)	Duration ± s.d.
Rat	1 −10	0·0136 ± 0·0038	<1·0	0·69 ± 0·25
Rabbit	0·01–0·1	2·60 ± 1·26	0·35 ± 0·21	0·66 ± 0·20
Cat	0·01–0·15	1·72 ± 0·46	<1·0	0·49 ± 0·14
Dog	0·03–0·1	2·5 ± 0·9	0·46 ± 0·07	0·50 ± 0·14
Baboon	0·02–0·1	0·83	—	0·46

From Buckett (1968).

activity was provided in the conventional tests such as reversal with neostigmine and absence of contracture in frog and avian muscle. The compound possesses some cardiac vagolytic action and it can release histamine in guinea pigs. Some anticholinesterase activity is also present.

3.3.2   Species sensitivity to neuromuscular blockers

The findings in Table 8 allow some speculation regarding species sensitivity. It has long been known that the nondepolarizing agent tubocurarine is more potent in the rat than in the cat (Goodman and Gilman, 1970), yet dacuronium is in all respects a nondepolarizing agent but much less potent in the rat than in other species. This led Derkx et al. (1971) to examine other nondepolarizing agents and it was found that indeed only tubocurarine showed greater potency in the rat and is not therefore typical of this class of blocker. However, the rat is extremely resistant to dacuronium bromide and this is unlikely to be due to metabolism in vivo, since the compound is even less active on the isolated phrenic nerve–diaphragm preparation of the rat. It is possible that the steroidal nucleus has some peculiar property in the rat since the highly active compound pancuronium bromide, having a potency of some five times that of tubocurarine in man, has less than the potency of tubocurarine in the rat (Buckett *et al.*, 1968). The particularly low sensitivity of the rat would be due to other effects of tubocurarine such as the release of histamine which might desensitize the motor end-plate in some way to the neuromuscular blocking actions of the drug. However, dacuronium bromide has one-third the potency of tubocurarine in releasing histamine to cause bronchoconstriction in the guinea pig, but is much less active in releasing histamine from the peritoneal mast cells in the rat. Results of experiments designed to illustrate the role of histamine in this regard could be extremely interesting.

3.3.3 *Cat muscle sensitivity to neuromuscular blockers*

In the cat tubocurarine is more effective in blocking slow-contracting muscles (Paton and Zaimis, 1951) whereas depolarizing agents are more effective in blocking fast-contracting muscles. The advent of the steroidal neuromuscular blockers has cast doubt on this categorical statement. For example, Bonta and Goorissen (1968) showed that pancuronium bromide produced a greater degree of neuromuscular block in the tibialis anterior muscle of the cat than in the soleus muscle. Dacuronium bromide has recently been shown (Marshall, 1973a) to be equi-active in the two muscles. Marshall (1973a) on the basis of findings not only with dacuronium bromide but also with stercuronium (**7**) and a new nonsteroidal blocker, fazadinium bromide, AH8165 (1,1'-azobis[3-methyl-2-phenyl-1*H*-imidazo-(1,2-a)pyridinium] dibromide) (**21**) (Brittain and Tyers, 1972) suggests

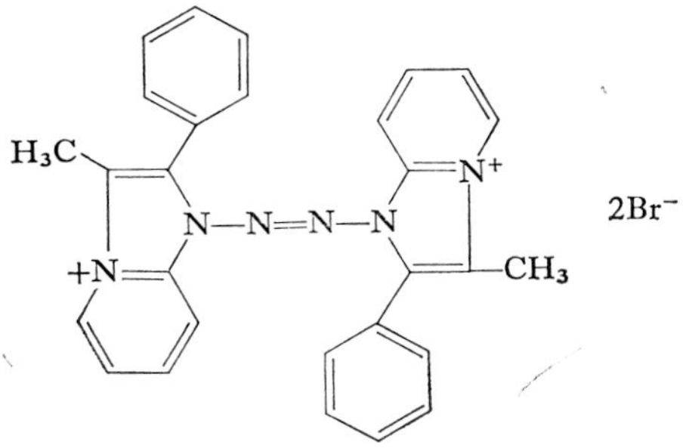

(21)

that the different susceptibilities of fast- and slow-contracting muscles is not satisfactory for classifying these drugs into depolarizing and non-depolarizing groups. In addition there is no relationship between inhibition of cat muscle acetylcholinesterase and blocking action so it has been postulated that the muscle selectivity is due to slight differences in the cholinoceptor configuration in the two muscles.

3.3.4 *Predictive models for duration of action*

Since the ideal short-acting nondepolarizing agent still appears elusive, more newly synthesized steroidal compounds are submitted for screening. Nevertheless the prediction of human activity from animal data in this seemingly relatively simple field of pharmacological action is as difficult as ever. Mushin and Mapleson (1964) in studying dipyrandium maintained that the monkey would be the optimum species for examination prior to man, in contrast to Bowman (1962) who recommended the use of the cat. The atypical behaviour of steroidal neuromuscular blocking agents in various muscles and various species has led Marshall (1973b) to study dacuronium bromide, pancuronium bromide and stercuronium iodide in the cat in some depth and to suggest that the slow-contracting soleus muscle may be a better model than the tibialis anterior for predicting duration of action in man. It is quite clear from the discussion above (section 3.3.2) that the rat is an unsatisfactory model for prediction either *in vitro* (phrenic nerve–diaphragm) or *in vivo*.

3.3.5 *Cardiovascular effects of dacuronium bromide*

Dacuronium bromide possesses some selective atropine-like anticholinergic activity which appears to be cardiac-specific, resulting in increases in heart rate and blood pressure (Buckett and Saxena, 1969). This activity appears at doses lower than those required for blockade of the neuromuscular junction. The cardioselective vagolytic action of dacuronium bromide has been confirmed (Marshall, 1973c) in anaesthetized cats in which the brady-cardia produced by vagal stimulation and by amechol was unaffected. Dacuronium bromide also shows weak sympathetic ganglion blocking activity but hypotension is not seen due to the masking of this action by the cardiac vagolytic effects. Sympathomimetic amine release such as that demonstrated with gallamine (Brown and Crout, 1970) has not been shown for dacuronium bromide at the present time.

3.3.6 *Clinical studies with dacuronium bromide*

Using an ingenious "isolated" human arm technique in which circulation was temporarily reduced by a pneumatic tourniquet at 200 mmHg, dacuronium bromide was studied in conscious volunteers (Feldman and Tyrrell, 1970). The muscle contraction of the adductor pollucis longus in response to supramaximal ulnar nerve stimulation showed that in the presence of dacuronium a block occurred which was reversed by edrophonium and during which post-tetanic facilitation was observed, thus classifying the drug as nondepolarizing in type. The duration was shorter than that of gallamine, but in clinical trials using full blocking dosage dacuronium bromide and gallamine were found to be similar with respect to potency, duration and cardiac vagolytic action (Norman and Katz, 1971). The tachycardia produced by dacuronium bromide was always marked in man. Another complication which arose was due to the action of the drug in inhibiting plasma cholinesterase, causing prolongation of suxamethonium to the extent, in one patient at least, of a 2-hour apnoea (Stovner, J., personal communication).

Thus dacuronium bromide, a drug which was unsatisfactory for clinical use, has been discussed here at some length. This was felt to be justified since it challenged some of the long-held textbook beliefs regarding neuro-muscular blocking agents, particularly with respect to species and muscle selectivity.

3.3.7 Dacuronium iodide

Dacuronium iodide was also prepared and examined pharmacologically. It was very similar to the bromide, although somewhat less potent as a neuromuscular blocking agent. It had greater propensity for histamine release and, as was observed frequently with the iodides of bisquaternary steroids, tended to be less stable on storage.

3.3.8 Org 6368 ($2\beta,16\beta$-dipiperidino-5α-androstan-3α-ol acetate dimetho-bromide) (22)

Since it was suggested that hydrolysis of the ester function at 3α in dacur-onium bromide was probably responsible for its short duration, yet the presence of a 17β-hydroxy group was probably responsible for the weakness of its action in man, perhaps because of nonspecific protein binding, then the absence of the 17β-hydroxyl might lead to a more potent drug. Org 6368 (22) was indeed more potent than tubocurarine with onset and recovery time in the cat similar to that of suxamethonium (Sugrue and Duff, 1973). It is nondepolarizing in nature and has ganglion-blocking and histamine-releasing actions quantitatively similar to dacuronium bromide. Slight hypertension and occasional tachycardia were also noted. In cats, Org 6368 is rapidly taken up by the liver with a consequently low circulating plasma concentration. How this metabolic disposition will affect clinical usage remains to be seen.

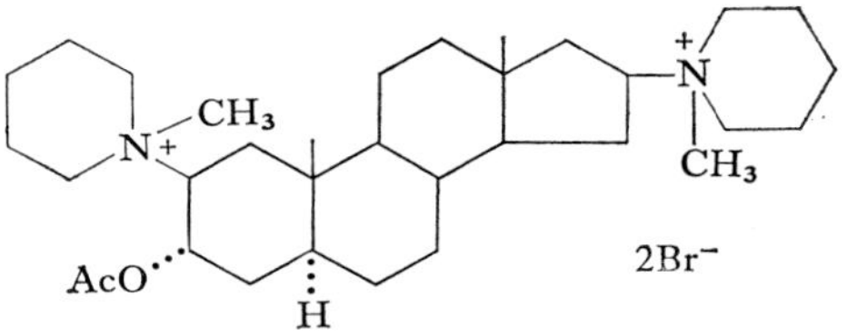

(22)

3.4 MISCELLANEOUS ANDROSTANES AND OTHER COMPOUNDS

An early attempt to utilize the steroid nucleus as a supporting structure for quaternary ammonium groups was made by Cavallani *et al.* (1951) who examined the dimethiodide of the bisdiethylaminoethyl ether of androst-5-ene-3,17-diol (23). The action of this compound was noted at $0{\cdot}1$ mg kg^{-1}

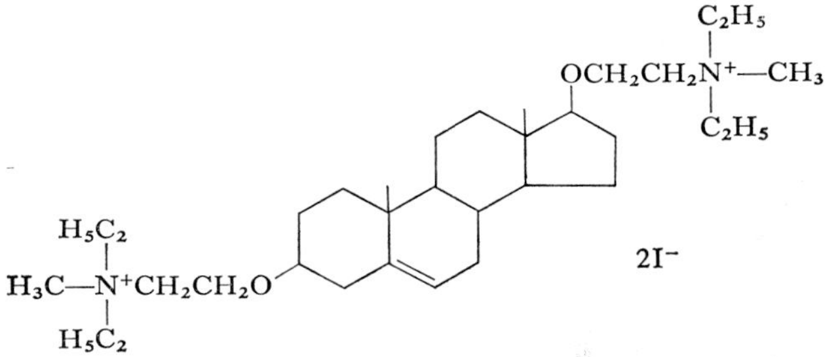

(23)

in dogs and was not antagonized by neostigmine, suggesting a depolarizing type of action. However, the compound antagonized acetylcholine on the frog rectus abdominis muscle which was indicative of nondepolarizing mode of action. No cardiovascular effects were noted in dogs at ten times the neuromuscular blocking dose but neither this compound, nor the oestradiol analogue, appear to have been studied further, probably because of the long duration of action.

A number of $2\beta,17\beta$-diamino-5α-androstan-$3\alpha,16\beta$-diols, acetates and diacetates have been described by Buckett *et al.* (1973), none of which proved to have potent action or short duration. The most active compound (24) was the isomer of pancuronium bromide, but it was less than one-tenth as active as the parent compound (17g). Other attempts in this area either to shorten duration or increase potency did not yield satisfactory compounds. Finally in order to confirm that the incorporation of an acetylcholine fragment within the ring was really essential, a compound with acetylcholine extra to the ring system, $3\beta,17\beta$-di(methyl-2′-acetoxyethylamino)-

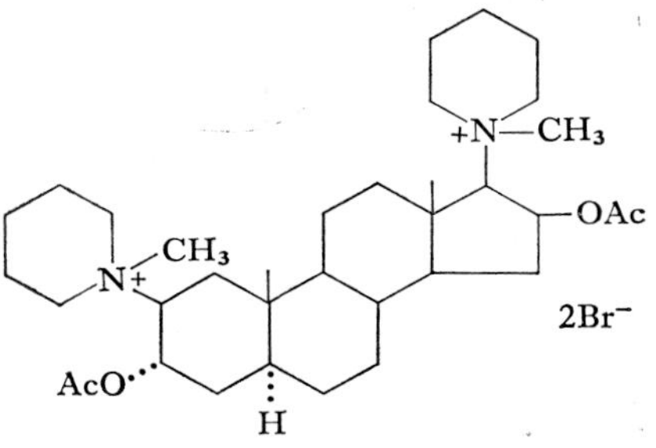

(24)

5α-androstane dimethobromide (25) was prepared and found to possess low potency. A further example of incorporation of the quaternary nitrogen

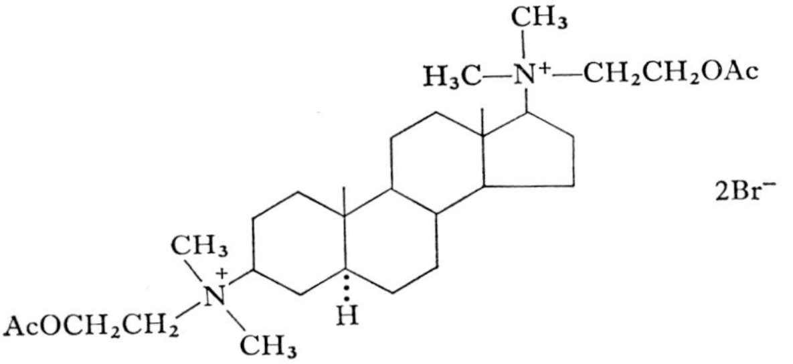

(25)

atoms within a *D*-homo-5α-androstane structure has been effected by Singh *et al.* (1972) who prepared 4,17a-dimethyl-4,17a-diaza-*D*-homo-5α-androstane dimethiodide (HS-342) (26). This compound has been the subject of extensive pharmacological investigations (Marshall, 1968; Marshall

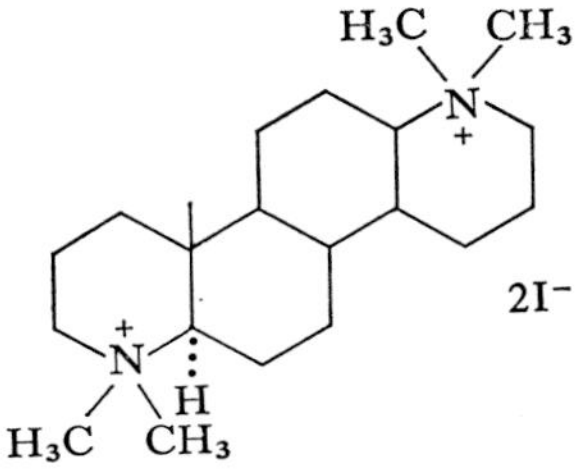

(26)

et al., 1972; 1973a; 1973b) and whilst having a potent action of short duration at the neuromuscular junction was not completely selective for the receptors at that site. It also possessed ganglionic blocking and cardiac vagolytic actions. The net effect on blood pressure was hypotensive. The anticholinesterase action of the drug was of a low order and the neuromuscular blocking action was characterized as nondepolarizing. The drug does not appear to have been investigated clinically.

Recently a steroid-related triterpenoid compound, the quillaite of choline iodide (27) has been described (Hamed and El-Gholmy, 1972) as being slow in onset, weaker and of longer duration than tubocurarine.

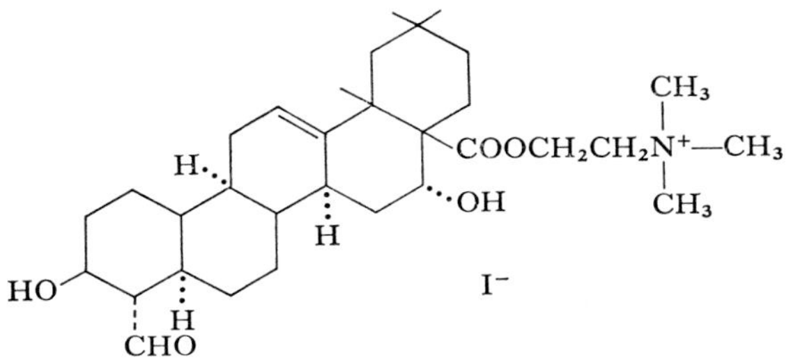

(27)

Its action appears to be mainly prejunctional and since it is not reversed by neostigmine it is not likely to be a nondepolarizing drug, yet it does in fact produce flaccid paralysis in avians.

An extremely potent natural product, a steroidal alkaloid, isolated from the Colombian arrow-poison frog (*Phyllobates aurotaenia*) and called batrachotoxin (28) (Märki and Witkop, 1963) is used as a pharmacological agent in the study of ion transport and nerve function. The alkaloid blocks neuromuscular transmission irreversibly by increasing the nerve membrane permeability to sodium. This increase in permeability also elicits many

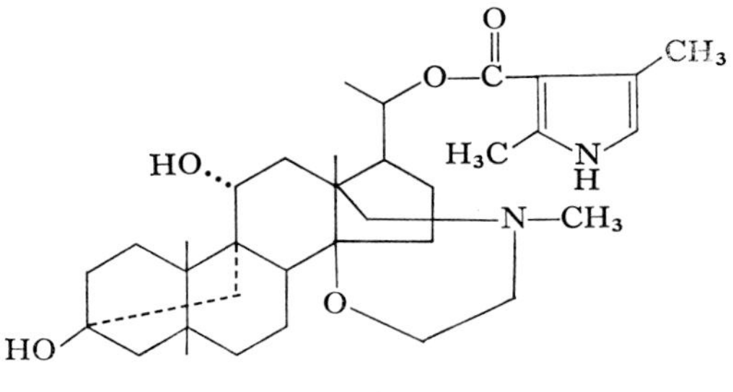

(28)

secondary phenomena both pre- and postjunctionally. This compound is unlikely to achieve any medical use so is precluded from further discussion here. The most recent review on batrachotoxin is by Albuquerque *et al.* (1971) and may be consulted by the interested reader.

4 Pancuronium bromide

4.1 INTRODUCTION

Pancuronium bromide (Pavulon®) is a bisquaternary ammonium steroidal compound (**17**g) of the series described by Buckett *et al.* (1973) which has been widely used to produce muscle relaxation of rapid onset and medium duration in clinical anaesthesia. It has little effect on the cardiovascular system, does not release histamine and, although a steroid, is free from hormonal activity.

4.2 CHEMISTRY

The background to this area has already been described in section 3.2. In the 2β-monoquaternary aminosteroid corresponding to pancuronium, the 2β-piperidino and 3α-acetoxy groups are almost certainly both pseudo-equatorial due to the conformation of ring A in twisted-boat form and it was believed that in this preferred conformation, which may be rigid due to steric compression of ring A substituents, the acetylcholine-like fragment resembles a specific molecular conformation of acetylcholine as it perhaps exists at the neuromuscular junction. The addition of a similar fragment at positions 16 and 17 in the androsterone nucleus gave pseudo-equatorial conformation in the 5-membered ring D. This appeared to be the optimal substitution for specific neuromuscular blocking activity of high potency.

Pancuronium bromide may be readily prepared in six stages from the naturally occurring steroid 5α-androst-2-en-17-one (Fig. 1), a preparation described in detail by Buckett *et al.* (1973). The infrared spectrum exhibits maxima at 3340 to 3380 cm^{-1} (quaternary nitrogen) and 1745 to 1760 cm^{-1} (acetate).

4.3 MOLECULAR STRUCTURE AND RECEPTOR INTERACTIONS

In an elegant X-ray crystallographic study Savage *et al.* (1971) have shown that the interonium distance (N$^+$---N$^+$) in pancuronium bromide is 11·08 Å and, although this distance was nearer 10 Å in less active isomers when calculated from molecular models, it cannot be said with any certainty that 11·08 Å is indeed the sole criterion for conferring potency and specificity since asymmetry is another governing factor. Other factors including the steric interactions in pancuronium bromide are such, when deduced from nmr spectra, that the molecule must possess a fairly rigid structure which

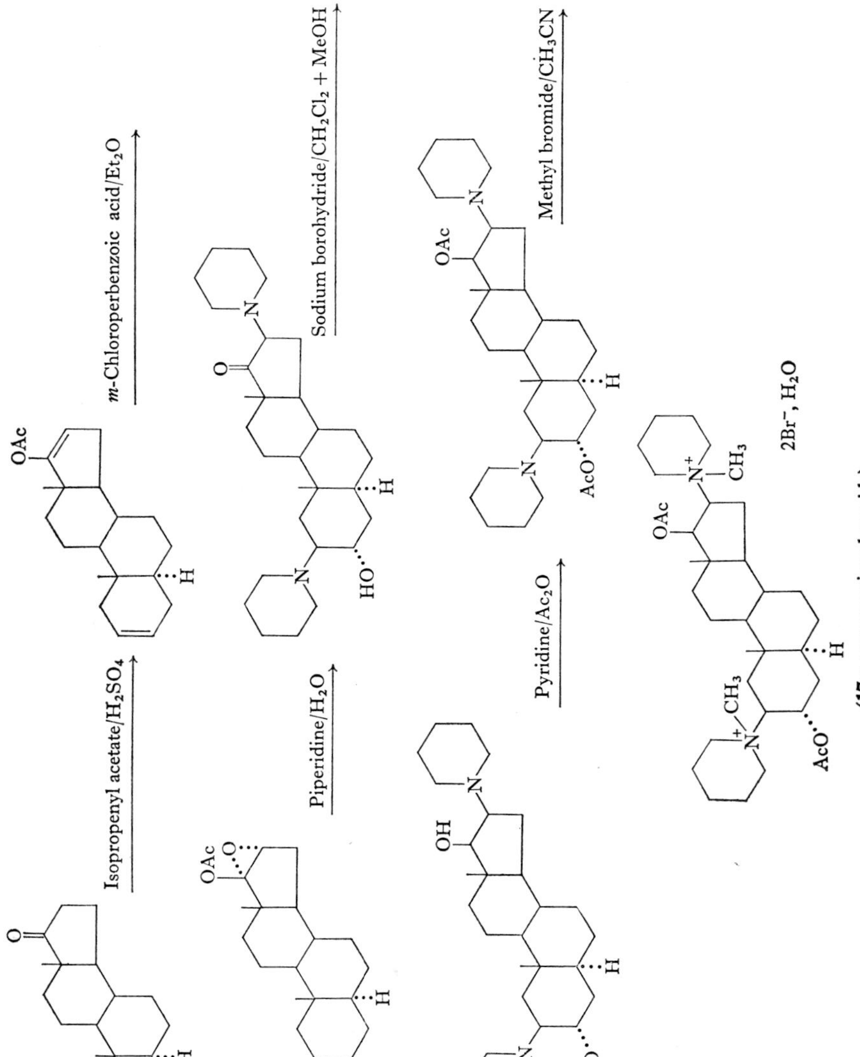

(**17***g*: pancuronium bromide)

FIG. 1. **Preparation of pancuronium bromide.**

may be optimal for attachment to a neuromuscular receptor site. Since optical isomers having one centre of asymmetry, for example noradrenaline, can differ markedly in potency and pharmacological action, it is worth noting that pancuronium bromide possesses no fewer than ten such asymmetric centres. Tubocurarine possesses only two centres of asymmetry.

The acetylcholine fragments in pancuronium bromide are fairly rigid from the evidence already mentioned and they present a *cis*-orientation of

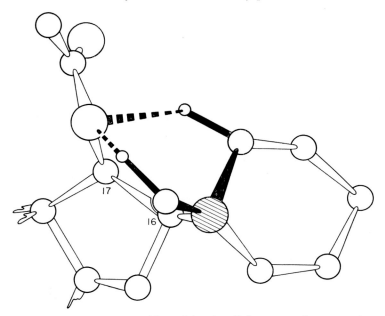

FIG. 2. The molecular packing of the ring *D* fragment of pancuronium.

both ester and quaternary ammonium head to the receptor. It has been suggested that unique hydrogen bonding systems, involving *quasi* six-ring formation ($C-C-\overset{+}{N}-C-H \text{---} OCOCH_3$) are formed within each of the acetylcholine-like fragments of the molecule. The hydrogen bonding in the ring *D* fragment (Fig. 2) involves two *quasi* six-membered rings and is more complex than that in the ring *A* acetylcholine fragment.

Intramolecular hydrogen bonding in acetylcholine has been suggested by Sutor (1963), but its existence has only recently been proved by the quantum theoretical study of the molecular electronic structure of acetylcholine (Beveridge and Radna, 1971). It may be concluded from the molecular structure studies that the more involved ring *D* substituents could well contribute more to the potency and duration of pancuronium bromide than those attached to ring A (Fig. 3). This conclusion has also been reached by Michoel and Kinget (1973) who have reported that the difference in rate constants for the 17- and 3-acetoxy groups confirms the molecular structure suggested above for these areas of the molecule.

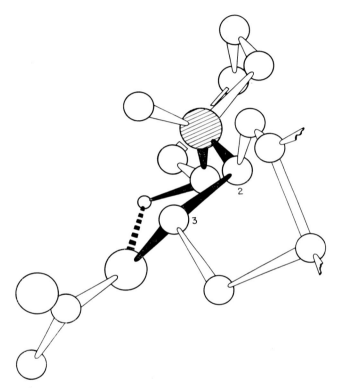

Fig. 3. The molecular packing of the ring A fragment of pancuronium.

4.4   ACTION OF PANCURONIUM BROMIDE AT THE NEUROMUSCULAR JUNCTION

The exact sites and modes of action of pancuronium at the neuromuscular junction have not been fully elucidated. It is clear, however, that it possesses, in common with other nondepolarizing agents, both prejunctional and post-junctional effects with relative potency differing according to species and preparation.

Pancuronium was first shown to be a potent neuromuscular blocking agent of medium duration of action in the anaesthetized cat sciatic-gastrocnemius preparation (Buckett *et al.*, 1968). In experiments where both nerve and muscle action potentials were recorded simultaneously, neuromuscular blocking doses of pancuronium of 0·01 to 0·02 mg kg^{-1} intravenously abolished the muscle action whereas potentials along the nerve were unaffected. During this block, direct stimulation of the muscle with electrodes caused normal contractions indicating lack of direct depressant effect on the muscle. These results define the action of pancuronium at the neuromuscular junction.

Evidence for a postjunctional action of pancuronium was gained from reduction of the sensitivity of the muscle to intra-arterial acetylcholine and the fact that the blockade due to pancuronium could be reversed by neostigmine, edrophonium and more recently pyridostigmine (Fogdall and Miller, 1973). The neuromuscular blockade was augmented by small doses of tubocurarine insufficient to cause a block alone. Potassium chloride and the depolarizing agent suxamethonium antagonized neuromuscular blockade due to pancuronium. These findings have been confirmed by many investigators using similar mammalian preparations (Marshall, 1968; Crul, 1970; Derkx et al., 1971). Species which exhibit muscle contracture in response to depolarizing agents do not show pancuronium to have such a mode of action. Thus acetylcholine-induced contracture of frog rectus abdominis muscle is abolished by pancuronium and the agent itself does not cause contracture of the muscle. In the hen pancuronium produces a flaccid paralysis in conscious animals and contracture is not demonstrated in anaesthetized preparations.

Recently more sophisticated studies have confirmed the postjunctional effects of pancuronium. For example, using an amphibian single fibre nerve muscle preparation, Karis and Gissen (1971) were able to show that the action potential in the nerve terminal was unchanged during pancuronium perfusion as was the transmembrane resting potential of the postjunctional membrane. In this study the response to acetylcholine was reduced confirming the postjunctional action. The evidence obtained by Galindo (1972) in the isolated rat diaphragm was also indicative of a predominantly postjunctional action. The resting potential of muscle fibres was not changed nor was the reversal potential of acetylcholine during the presence of pancuronium. The strength of muscular contraction was reduced. In contrast to tubocurarine, pancuronium did not affect the frequency of miniature end-plate potentials (mepp) although their amplitude was reduced. The depression of end-plate potential (epp) amplitude was depressed by pancuronium in a very specific fashion to give a double peak unlike other agents which produce a single peak. This makes calculations on transmitter output and mobilization somewhat inconsistent, a factor not apparent from work in the cat (Blaber, 1973). In the rat therefore pancuronium blocks neuromuscular transmission mainly by depressing

TABLE 9

Presynaptic effects of pancuronium and tubocurarine

Parameter	Species and preparation	Effect of tubocurarine	Reference	Effect of pancuronium	Reference
Available acetylcholine store	rat pnd	reduced	Hubbard *et al.* (1969)	reduced	Blaber (1973)
	cat tenuiss	reduced at higher concentration	Blaber (1973)		
Acetylcholine mobilization rate	rat pnd	reduced	Galindo (1972)	reduced	Blaber (1973)
	cat tenuiss	reduced	Blaber (1973)		
Spontaneous release of quanta (mepp frequency)	rat pnd	reduced	Galindo (1972)	not affected	Galindo (1972)
Mean quantum size (mepp amplitude)	rat pnd	reduced	Hubbard *et al.* (1969)	reduced	Galindo (1972)
	cat tenuiss	reduced	Blaber (1973)	reduced	Blaber (1973)
Mean quantal content of first epp	rat pnd	reduced	Galindo (1972)	inconclusive	Galindo (1972)
	cat tibialis	reduced	Blaber and Goode (1968)		
	cat tenuiss	increased at low, no effect at high concentration	Blaber (1973)	reduced	Blaber (1973)
Fractional release of acetylcholine	cat tenuiss	reduced	Blaber (1973)	not affected	Blaber (1973)
Post tetanic repetitive activity	cat soleus	reduced	Standaert (1964)	reduced	Sohn and Aldrete (1971)
Presynaptic membrane potential	rat pnd	increased	Galindo (1972)	not affected	Galindo (1972)

pnd, phrenic nerve-diaphragm.
tenuiss, tenuissimus nerve-muscle.

postjunctional receptors. This may therefore account for the weak potency of pancuronium (lower than tubocurarine) in the rat (Buckett *et al.*, 1968). It is clear that tubocurarine, of all known neuromuscular blockers, is most potent in this species (Derkx *et al.*, 1971). Using ^{14}C-labelled pancuronium in the mouse, Waser (1973) has shown that a high concentration of radioactivity is seen at the motor endplates, where the postsynaptic blockade occurs. The number of molecules (5×10^6 at a dose of 0.15 μg g^{-1}) was similar to values obtained with other nondepolarizing blocking agents saturating the membrane, but uptake is somewhat slower and release takes longer. This is a reflection of this species-dependent long duration of action so it would be of great interest to see whether end-plate uptake and release rate in other species, such as the cat, could be correlated with its shorter duration of action in that species and in man.

It seems then that a prejunctional action of pancuronium (Table 9) could well be an important determinant of its high potency in other species, particularly the cat. The neural repetitive activity generated in the motor nerve terminal when it is reached by single stimuli after a period of high frequency stimulation is markedly affected by pancuronium which depresses this post-tetanic potentiation in subneuromuscular blocking doses (Sohn and Aldrete, 1971) or during a partial neuromuscular block (Buckett *et al.*, 1968).

Other evidence for the prejunctional action of pancuronium comes from work on facilitation of twitch height by anticholinesterase drugs. Marshall (1968) and Sohn and Aldrete (1971) have demonstrated antagonism by subneuromuscular blocking doses of pancuronium to neostigmine and edrophonium-induced facilitation in the cat tibialis and soleus as well as in the hen. In addition suxamethonium facilitation and also muscle fasciculations can be prevented by small doses of pancuronium, a property of the drug which is utilized clinically. Other studies with neostigmine and pancuronium using cat soleus muscle (Bowman and Webb, 1972) show pancuronium selectivity to depress twitch augmentation and muscle repetitive firing in doses that allowed fasciculation and antidromic ventral root repetition to continue. In contrast tubocurarine preferentially blocked muscle fasciculation and its associated electrical activity in nerve, a property believed to be more related to the affinity of tubocurarine for neuronal receptors, which is reflected in its ganglionic blocking potency. Using a cut-fibre preparation of isolated cat tenuissimus muscle, Blaber (1973) has provided evidence for prejunctional actions of pancuronium. Pancuronium, like tubocurarine, reduces the readily available acetylcholine stores (or primary pool) which is then replaced from a secondary pool at a slower rate under the influence of these drugs. The mean quantum size of acetylcholine reflected by mepp amplitude is similarly reduced. In response to stimulation the quantal content of acetylcholine in the first epp is reduced by pancuronium but not by tubocurarine. Pancuronium was without effect on fractional release (the fraction of stores released by the first impulse) although tubocurarine depressed it. These results essentially support the findings in frogs of Gergis et al. (1972) and Dretchen et al. (1972) that pancuronium blocks the release of acetylcholine in concentrations that effect muscle blockade. These authors believe that in the frog the action of pancuronium is predominantly on the nerve terminal, since at lower concentrations pancuronium releases acetylcholine from the presynaptic nerve terminal. The mechanism of this acetylcholine release is not known, but it is not related to synthesis of the transmitter or to the nerve action potential since both hemicholinium and tetrodotoxin are without effect. Calcium must be present for pancuronium to cause this release of acetylcholine from resting nerve. It is of interest to note that the potency of pancuronium in the frog is also low compared with other species (Buckett et al., 1968). The relevance of these findings in application to clinical medicine remains obscure at the present time.

In studies on the importance of the prejunctional depolarizing action of acetylcholine, Bowman and Webb (1972) obtained results to show that pancuronium produced a waning of tetanic tension only during a considerable degree of neuromuscular blockade, confirming the results of Buckett et al. (1968), in contrast to tubocurarine which causes rapid waning even under slight neuromuscular blockade. This is interpreted once more as the result of a greater affinity of pancuronium for muscle receptors, i.e. a postjunctional predominance, and similar findings with tetanic stimulation have indeed been secured clinically (Hunter, 1970).

Pancuronium bromide therefore possesses both pre- and postjunctional actions at the neuromuscular junction. It appears probable from work on mammalian systems and from clinical evidence that its main action is postjunctional due to a somewhat greater affinity for muscle receptors. The interesting findings from experiments designed to study prejunctional actions must always be interpreted with considerable caution, care being taken in assessing species, experimental design and particularly the concentration of drugs and ionic solutions used. The uncertainty as to the exact locus of action of pancuronium at the neuromuscular junction will doubtless spur on further investigators to elucidate this problem. Interactions with other prejunctionally acting drugs used in other fields may also yield interesting information, for example lithium carbonate, currently in wide use in psychiatry, acts by reducing presynaptic acetylcholine release, so that when pancuronium is administered a prolonged neuromuscular blockade may be observed (Borden et al., 1974).

The importance of the species used in this type of experiment cannot be over-emphasized. The rabbit, cat and dog are similarly sensitive to pancuronium (Buckett et al., 1968) whereas mouse and man have a similar but lower sensitivity to the drug (Baird and Reid, 1967). Individual muscles within one species can also differ in their sensitivity to neuromuscular blocking drugs and pancuronium has similar actions on both soleus and tibialis muscles, unlike tubocurarine and other nondepolarizing agents which are more active on the soleus muscle, and suxamethonium and depolarizing agents which more readily block the tibialis in the anaesthetized cat (Bonta and Goorisen, 1968). In a pithed rat preparation pancuronium was less potent than tubocurarine and did not show selectivity for either tibialis or soleus muscles (Clanachan and Muir, 1972).

The specificity of pancuronium as a nondepolarizing neuromuscular blocking agent is suggested by the absence of anti-acetylcholine or atropine-like action on the guinea-pig ileum, together with low ganglionic blocking potency in a variety of preparations (Buckett et al., 1968; Marshall, 1968). It is possible also that the high potency of this compound is a contributing factor to its specificity.

4.5   PHARMACOLOGY AND DRUG INTERACTIONS

General pharmacological studies with pancuronium have centred on its action on the cardiovascular system, since it is on this system that the drug differs most clearly from tubocurarine. The conclusion from animal work is that pancuronium can cause a marginal increase in heart rate and arterial blood pressure (Smith et al., 1970; Saxena and Bonta, 1970; Sharma, 1970). In very high doses it may have a selective cardiac vagolytic action, since the effects of vagal stimulation, as well as the negative inotropic and chronotropic effects of cholinergic drugs are attenuated, whereas the peripheral vascular effects of such drugs are not affected by pancuronium (Bonta et al., 1968; Saxena and Bonta, 1970).

The absence of a hypotensive effect with pancuronium is due to its low ganglionic blocking potency and also to its absence of histamine-releasing propensity. Thus, bronchoconstriction in guinea pigs, hypotension in ganglion-blocked cats, increase in circulating histamine in rabbits and histamine release from mast cells of the rat were all absent after exposure to pancuronium (Buckett et al., 1968; Buckett and Frisk-Holmberg, 1970). The absence of free hydroxyl groups in the molecule is probably the most significant factor, since similar steroids with one free hydroxyl group (dacuronium; 20) or two hydroxyl groups (17a) release histamine. The fact that Org 6368 (22) releases histamine (Sugrue and Duff, 1973) to a similar extent to dacuronium suggests that metabolic hydroxylation or rapid hydrolysis of the 3-acetate may occur.

Pancuronium is free from endocrinological actions when tested in hormone screening tests in rats at 0·3 mg kg^{-1} subcutaneously (Visser and van der Vies, 1968), an unsurprising finding in view of the hydrophilicity of the molecule. It is possible that pancuronium may have some action in the adrenal gland in releasing both adrenaline and noradrenaline from the adrenal medulla. Nana et al. (1973) suggest that this may be the mechanism which is responsible for the slight rise in blood pressure and pulse rate after pancuronium administration. At least these findings were obtained with neuromuscular blocking doses and not after the large doses necessary to demonstrate a cardiac vagolytic effect in animals (Saxena and Bonta, 1970) and as such lend credibility to the action of pancuronium in releasing medullary neurohormones.

Experimental halothane-adrenaline arrhythmias in the dog are reduced in severity and duration by pancuronium (Sharma, 1970), so this led to an investigation on interactions between pancuronium and beta-adrenergic blocking agents such as propranolol, alprenolol and practolol. Potentiation of the neuromuscular blockade on the isolated rat phrenic-nerve-diaphragm preparation was found (Saini and Sharma, 1971) but these findings have not been extended to in vivo experiments hence their clinical relevance is open to doubt. Other investigations with pancuronium in the presence of halothane have shown that the latter reinforces the neuromuscular blockade, but that the hypotensive effect of halothane is not potentiated by pancuronium but rather the reverse (Bonta and Buckett, 1969). Tubocurarine on the other hand can cause marked blood pressure falls in the presence of halothane. Ether and thiopentone can also potentiate the neuromuscular blocking activity of pancuronium. Pancuronium can prevent neuromuscular blockade due to decamethonium on the rat phrenic diaphragm (Foldes and Pan, 1969). Some antibiotics such as streptomycin can potentiate the neuromuscular blockade due to nondepolarizing agents and occasionally this can cause clinical concern as with pancuronium and polymyxin-B (Fogdall and Miller, 1974).

4.6   TOXICOLOGY AND METABOLISM

4.6.1   Toxicity studies

The acute lethality of pancuronium bromide is high (Table 10) due to its pharmacological action of neuromuscular blockade and subsequent respiratory failure. It is therefore important to be aware that the acute toxicity of pancuronium bromide when administered to artificially ventilated animals is in fact very low indeed. For example, in anaesthetized cats under artificial respiration, up to 25 000 times the neuromuscular blocking dose could be tolerated (Buckett et al., 1968) and in dogs up to 600 times the

TABLE 10

The acute lethality of pancuronium bromide in various species

Species	Route	LD_{50} (mg kg^{-1})
Mouse	intravenous	0·047 (0·045–0·050)
Mouse	intraperitoneal	0·152 (0·144–0·160)
Mouse	subcutaneous	0·167 (0·158–0·175)
Mouse	oral	21·9 (19·0 –25·2)
Rat	intravenous	0·153 (0·136–0·172)
Rabbit	intravenous	0·016 (0·015–0·018)

neuromuscular blocking dose acutely and 1500 times the dose on fourteen occasions were well tolerated (Speight and Avery, 1972). Chronic studies by infusion of large doses of pancuronium bromide for a month in dogs showed no pathology of significance apart from mild perivascular eosinophilic infiltration in the liver occurring in one dog. Teratogenic studies in rats and rabbits did not yield any evidence of foetal abnormalities, although as with all drugs care should be exercised in the use of pancuronium bromide in pregnant patients.

4.6.2 Absorption and distribution

Pancuronium bromide is only used by intravenous injection, so naturally all pharmacokinetic studies have been based on this route of administration. Clinical studies on the correlation between the dose of pancuronium required and plasma protein levels imply that no significant binding to either albumin or globulin occurs (Stovner et al., 1971). This has been explained on the basis of the absence of free hydroxyl groups in the molecule, which are associated with globulin association, and the absence of charge-dissipating quaternization, such as found in alcuronium, which precludes albumin affinity. It has also been shown recently, using in vitro microdialysis, that at low concentration (0·03 to 0·3 μg ml^{-1}) only 20 per cent pancuronium bromide was protein bound and at 10 μg ml^{-1} this was decreased to 6 per cent (Waser, 1973).

The distribution of pancuronium has been investigated using ^{14}C-labelled material in mice (Waser, 1973) and in dogs (Speight and Avery, 1972). The study in mice utilized the autoradiographic technique and showed that the distribution of radioactivity in the aqueous compartment of the mouse body was very rapid with urinary elimination starting immediately. The only early tissue binding takes place in various cartilaginous areas and radioactivity then accumulates in the liver through six hours. It is this long time in the liver which has precluded human studies with ^{14}C-pancuronium. Interestingly, rapid accumulation also occurs in the adrenal cortex but not in the adrenal medulla of the mouse, so the role of endogenous catecholamines in the production of the slight tachycardia seen clinically may be questionable in respect to the potential releasing activity of pancuronium in the adrenal medulla. In dogs uptake into liver and kidney is the major tissue disposition, although pituitary, adrenals, spleen and heart also contained high levels of radioactivity through 24 hours.

Transplacental passage of pancuronium bromide is evidently slight. It was not detected in the mouse (Waser, 1973) using autoradiography, but with conventional radioactivity counts the ^{14}C-pancuronium could be demonstrated on foetuses of the rat after intravenous administration maternally. From a group of twenty patients undergoing Caesarean section, eleven offspring showed traces of pancuronium after maternal injection (Spiers and Sim, 1972) but were clinically satisfactory. This study and that of Forgacs (1970) showed the clinical suitability of pancuronium for this indication.

4.6.3 *Metabolism and excretion*

With the recent advent of a relatively simple quantitative method for the determination of pancuronium bromide and its metabolites (Kersten *et al.*, 1973), a number of meaningful studies on the metabolic fate of pancuronium in cats (Agoston *et al.*, 1973a) and in man (Agoston *et al.*, 1973b) have appeared, supplementing the earlier reports using ^{14}C-labelled pancuronium in dogs (Speight and Avery, 1972) and in the isolated canine liver (Strunin *et al.*, 1972). The general pattern (Table 11) which is emerging for man, dog and cat is that the major metabolic pathway is excretion of unchanged pancuronium bromide in the urine with a secondary pathway via the liver and the bile. Biotransformation does occur, mainly to the 3-hydroxy compound (**17**c) but with traces of dacuronium (**17**f) and the diol (**17**a) having been observed in the cat. The rat differs in that no biliary excretion is effected by this species (Meijer and Weitering, 1970), yet a further example of the difference in handling characteristics of this species with respect to aminosteroids.

The disappearance of pancuronium from the plasma after intravenous administration in man (Agoston *et al.*, 1973b) is due to an early rapid distribution phase (half life of less than five minutes) in which pharmacological actions can be detected at 0·6 minutes and maximum neuromuscular blockade at 2·4 minutes (Norman *et al.*, 1970). This is followed by a slower decline in plasma levels (half-life of 7 to 13 minutes) presumably dependent upon redistribution and excretion in which plasma protein

TABLE 11

The metabolites of pancuronium bromide and their distribution in certain species

Metabolites	Metabolic and excretory pathway in:		
	Man[a]	Dog[b]	Cat[c]
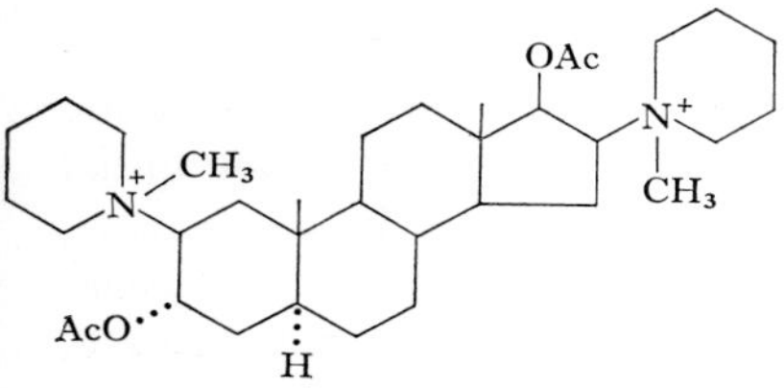 (17g: pancuronium)	Major (urine, bile)	Major (urine, bile)	Major (urine, liver, bile)
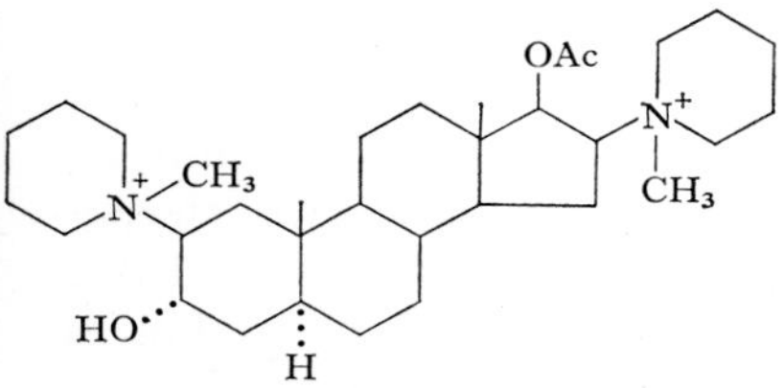 (17c)	Minor (urine, bile)	Minor (liver)	Minor (urine, liver, bile)
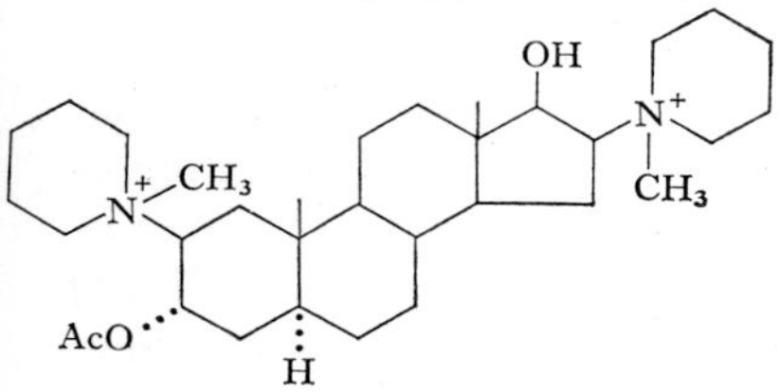 (17f: dacuronium)	Not detected (urine, bile)	Not detected (liver)	Minor (urine, liver, bile)
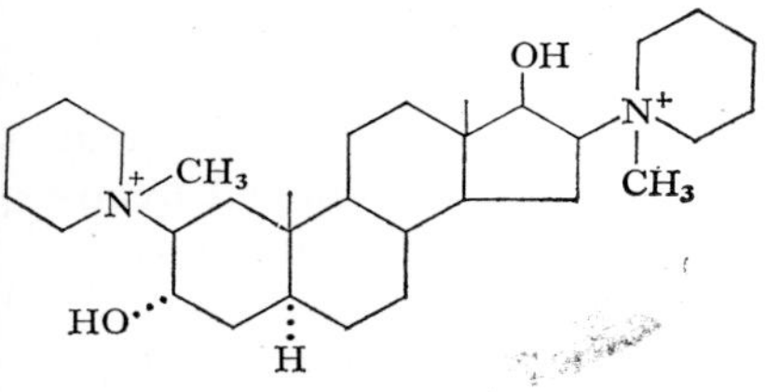 (17a)	Not detected (urine, bile)	Traces (liver)	Traces (urine, liver, bile)

[a] Agoston et al. (1973b).   [b] van der Veen (1971).   [c] Agoston et al. (1973a).

binding does not seem to be an important factor (Stovner *et al.*, 1971). Final elimination is represented by the third phase (half-life of 108–147 minutes). Essentially similar findings obtained in dogs (van der Veen, 1971), although a two-compartment elimination takes place in cats (Agoston *et al.*, 1973a).

4.7   CLINICAL STATUS

The neuromuscular blocking activity of pancuronium bromide was demonstrated first in man by Baird and Reid (1967) using an electromyographic recording method. Many subsequent clinical studies confirmed the initial clinical finding as well as providing evidence for lack of histamine release, minimal ganglion blockade and consequent cardiovascular stability. Such clinical evidence has been reviewed recently in detail (Speight and Avery, 1972; and references cited).

In clinical usage pancuronium is about five times as potent as tubocurarine (Norman *et al.*, 1970) with a more rapid onset of action (Sellick, 1968) and more rapid reversal (Baird, 1969). Stovner and Lund (1970), in experiments utilizing the loss of grip strength in conscious volunteers, showed that in man the dose-response line for pancuronium was steeper than for tubocurarine, so that at increasing levels of relaxation the relative potency of pancuronium will increase. It has been pointed out by Foldes (1972) that the claimed faster kinetics may not hold when doses equipotent with other relaxants are in fact used, but it is the lower side-effect incidence of pancuronium which engenders confidence in using higher doses than may be required for adequate muscle relaxation. The duration of action is similar to that shown by tubocurarine and there is no cumulation following incremental doses of one-quarter the initial dose. The occasional increases in pulse rate and arterial blood pressure are dose related. Foldes *et al.* (1971) using 0.04 mg kg^{-1} pancuronium intravenously found no significant changes in pulse rate or blood pressure, but Kelman and Kennedy (1970) reported significant increases in pulse rate, arterial blood pressure, cardiac output and stroke volume after 0.07 mg kg^{-1} pancuronium. Peripheral vascular resistance is unchanged. The absence of histamine release and hence of bronchospasm make pancuronium suitable for use in asthmatics and bronchitics, and the absence of ganglion blockade and subsequent hypotension make for good cardiovascular stability, a factor of importance in "poor risk" and geriatric patients.

The clinical status therefore of pancuronium at the present time is perhaps suitably summarized by Foldes (1972) who states: "It stands to reason to select pancuronium for the production of surgical relaxation in all patients in whom there is no special indication for the use of another relaxant."

5 Conclusions

The aminosteroids have yielded many interesting compounds with potential therapeutic applications (see Buckett, 1972, for review) not least of which have been the steroidal neuromuscular blocking agents reviewed here in detail. From this area has emerged a clinically useful agent, pancuronium bromide, which has superseded the older neuromuscular blocking drugs mainly because of its lack of side effects. An explanation of the specificity of pancuronium has been offered, based on recent chemical and pharmacological studies. Nevertheless the seemingly impossible objective of a nondepolarizing neuromuscular blocking agent having a duration of action as short as that of the depolarizing agent suxamethonium remains chemically as elusive as ever, if indeed such a drug will ever be pharmacologically possible. Approaches to this objective have been made using the steroidal neuromuscular blocking agents but at best the duration of action has been twice that desired and the action has usually been coupled with cardiovascular and other side effects which administration of higher intravenous doses of aminosteroid generally brings. These derivatives have usually been less potent than the longer-acting agents such as pancuronium. It is always possible that future research may allow utilization of the steroid nucleus, perhaps in the presence of some as yet undefined metabolic process, in achieving this desired anaesthesiological goal.

References

Agoston, S., Kersten, U. W. and Meijer, D. K. F. (1973a). *Acta Anaesthesiologica Scandinavica*, **17**, 129.

Agoston, S., Vermeer, G. A., Kersten, U. W. and Meijer, D. K. F. (1973b). *Acta Anaesthesiologica Scandinavica*, **17**, 267.

Alauddin, M., Caddy, B., Lewis, J. J., Martin-Smith, M. and Sugrue, M. F. (1965). *Journal of Pharmacy and Pharmacology*, **17**, 55.

Albuquerque, E. X., Daly, J. W. and Witkop, B. (1971). *Science*, **172**, 995.

Baird, W. L. M. (1969). Abstracts of the Symposium International de l'Anesthésie at Ostend, April 17–20.

Baird, W. L. M. and Reid, A. M. (1967). *British Journal of Anaesthesia*, **39**, 775.

Bamford, D. G., Biggs, D. F., Davis, M. and Parnell, E. W. (1967). *British Journal of Pharmacology and Chemotherapy*, **30**, 194.

Bamford, D. G., Biggs, D. F., Davis, M. and Parnell, E. W. (1971). *Journal of Pharmacy and Pharmacology*, **23**, 595.

Bertho, A. (1944). *Annalen*, **555**, 214.

Beveridge, D. S. and Radna, R. J. (1971). *Journal of the American Chemical Society*, **93**, 3739.

Biggs, R. S., Davis, M. and Wien, R. (1964). *Experientia*, **20**, 119.

Blaber, L. C. (1973). *British Journal of Pharmacology*, **47**, 109.

Blaber, L. C. and Goode, J. W. (1968). *International Journal of Neuropharmacology*, **7**, 429.

Blanpin, O. and Bretaudeau, J. (1961). *Comptes Rendus de la Société Biologique de Paris*, **155**, 878.

Bonta, I. L. and Buckett, W. R. (1969). *Acta Physiologica et Pharmacologica Neerlandica*, **15**, 392.

Bonta, I. L. and Goorisen, E. M. (1968). *European Journal of Pharmacology*, **4**, 303.

Bonta, I. L., Goorisen, E. M. and Derkx, F. H. (1968). *European Journal of Pharmacology*, **4**, 83.

Borden, H., Clarke, M. T. and Katz, H. (1974). *Canadian Anaesthetists Society Journal*, **21**, 79.

Bowman, W. C. (1962). *In* "Progress in Medicinal Chemistry" (Eds G. P. Ellis and G. B. West), vol. 2, p. 88. Butterworths, London.

Bowman, W. C. and Webb, S. N. (1972). *In* "Neuromuscular Blocking and Stimulating Agents" (Ed. J. Cheymol), vol. 2, chapter 16. International Encyclopedia of Pharmacology and Therapeutics, Section 14, pp. 427–502. Pergamon Press, Oxford.

Brittain, R. T. and Tyers, M. B. (1972). *British Journal of Pharmacology*, **45**, 158P.

Brown, B. R. and Crout, J. R. (1970). *Journal of Pharmacology and Experimental Therapeutics*, **172**, 266.

Buckett, W. R. (1968). Unpublished data.

Buckett, W. R. (1972). *In* "Advances in Steroid Biochemistry and Pharmacology", vol. 3, 39–65. (Eds M. H. Briggs and G. Christie) Academic Press, London and New York.

Buckett, W. R. and Bonta, I. L. (1966). *Federation Proceedings*, **25**, 718.

Buckett, W. R. and Frisk-Holmberg, M. (1970). *British Journal of Pharmacology*, **40**, 165P.

Buckett, W. R., Hewett, C. L. and Savage, D. S. (1967). *Chimica Therapeutica*, **2**, 186.

Buckett, W. R., Hewett, C. L. and Savage, D. S. (1973). *Journal of Medicinal Chemistry*, **16**, 1116.

Buckett, W. R., Marjoribanks, C. E. B., Marwick, F. A. and Morton, M. B. (1968). *British Journal of Pharmacology and Chemotherapy*, **32**, 671.

Buckett, W. R. and Saxena, P. R. (1969). Abstracts of the 4th International Congress on Pharmacology, Basel, p. 420.

Burn, J. H. (1914). *Journal of Pharmacology and Experimental Therapeutics*, **6**, 305.

Busfield, D., Child, K. J., Clarke, A. J., Davis, B. and Dodds, M. G. (1968). *British Journal of Pharmacology and Chemotherapy*, **32**, 609.

Cavallini, G., Ferrari, W., Montegazza, P. and Massarini, E. (1951). *Il Farmaco Scienza e Tecnica (Pavia)*, **6**, 815.

Clanachan, A. S. and Muir, T. C. (1972). *British Journal of Pharmacology*, **46**, 514.

Crul, J. F. (1970). *In* "Progress in Anaesthesiology" (Ed. T. Boulton), p. 418. Excerpta Medica, Amsterdam.

Derkx, F. H. M., Bonta, I. L. and Lagendijk, A. (1971). *European Journal of Pharmacology*, **16**, 105.

Dretchen, K. L., Sokoll, M. D., Gergis, S. D. and Long, J. P. (1972). *European Journal of Pharmacology*, **20**, 46.

Everett, A. J., Lowe, L. A. and Wilkinson, J. (1970). *Chemical Communications*, 1020.

Feldman, S. A. and Tyrrell, M. F. (1970). *Anaesthesia*, **25**, 349.

Fogdall, R. P. and Miller, R. D. (1973). *Anesthesiology*, **39**, 504.

Fogdall, R. P. and Miller, R. D. (1974). *Anesthesiology*, **40**, 84.

Foldes, F. F. (1972). *Drugs*, **4**, 153.

Foldes, F. F. and Pan, T. H. (1969). Unpublished data.

Foldes, F. F., Klonymus, D. H., Maisel, W., Sciammas, F. and Pan, T. (1971). *Anesthesiology*, **35**, 496.

Forgacs, I. (1970). Abstracts 3rd European Congress on Anaesthesia, Prague, p. 41.

Galindo, A. (1972). *Science*, **178**, 753.

Gergis, S. D., Dretchen, K. L., Sokoll, M. D. and Long, J. P. (1972). *Proceedings of the Society for Experimental Biology and Medicine*, **139**, 74.

Hamed, M. I. and El-Gholmy, Z. (1972). *Arzneimittel-Forschung*, **22**, 2133.

Hespe, W. and Wieriks, J. (1971). *Biochemical Pharmacology*, **20**, 1213.

Hewett, C. L. and Savage, D. S. (1968). *Journal of the Chemical Society*, *C*, 1134.

Hubbard, J. I., Wilson, D. F. and Miyamoto, M. (1969). *Nature, London*, **223**, 531.

Hunter, A. R. (1970). *Proceedings of the Royal Society of Medicine*, **63**, 699.

Janot, M., Lainé, F. and Goutarel, R. (1960). *Annales Pharmaceutiques Françaises*, **18**, 673.

Janot, M., Lainé, F., Khuong-Huu, Q. and Goutarel, R. (1962). *Bulletin de la Société Chimique de France*, 111.

Karis, J. H. and Gissen, A. J. (1971). *Anesthesiology*, **35**, 149.

Kelman, G. R. and Kennedy, B. R. (1970). *British Journal of Pharmacology*, **40**, 567P.

Kersten, U. W., Meijer, D. K. F. and Agoston, S. (1973). *Clinica Chimica Acta*, **44**, 59.

Khuong Huu-Lainé, F. and Pinto-Scognamiglio, W. (1964). *Archives Intérnationales de Pharmacodynamie et de Thérapie*, **147**, 209.

Koelle, G. B. (1970). *In* "The Pharmacological Basis of Therapeutics" (Eds L. S. Goodman and A. Gilman), p. 607. Macmillan, New York.

Le Men, J., Kan, C. and Beugelmans, R. (1963). *Bulletin de la Société Chimique de France*, 597.

Lewis, J. J., Martin-Smith, M., Muir, T. C. and Ross, H. H. (1967). *Journal of Pharmacy and Pharmacology*, **19**, 502.

Märki, F. and Witkop, B. (1963). *Experientia*, **19**, 329.

Marshall, I. G. (1968). PhD Thesis, University of Strathclyde, Glasgow.

Marshall, I. G. (1973a). *European Journal of Pharmacology*, **21**, 299.

Marshall, I. G. (1973b). Unpublished data.

Marshall, I. G. (1973c). *Journal of Pharmacy and Pharmacology*, **25**, 530.

Marshall, I. G., Paul, D. and Singh, H. (1972). *Journal of Pharmacy and Pharmacology*, **24**, Supplement 146P.

Marshall, I. G., Paul, D. and Singh, H. (1973a). *Journal of Pharmacy and Pharmacology*, **25**, 441.

Marshall, I. G., Paul, D. and Singh, H. (1973b). *European Journal of Pharmacology*, **22**, 129.

Martin-Smith, M. (1971). *In* "Drug Design" (Ed. E. J. Ariëns), vol. 2, p. 505. Academic Press, New York and London.

Meijer, D. K. F. and Weitering, J. G. (1970). *European Journal of Pharmacology*, **10**, 283.

Michoel, A. and Kinget, R. (1973). Abstracts *Féderation Internationale de Pharmaceutique* meeting, Stockholm, p. 232.

Mushin, W. W. and Mapleson, W. W. (1964). *British Journal of Anaesthesia*, **36**, 761.

Nana, A., Cardan, E. and Domokos, M. (1973). *Acta Anaesthesiologica Scandinavica*, **17**, 83.

Norman, J. and Katz, R. L. (1971). *British Journal of Anaesthesia*, **43**, 313.

Norman, J., Katz, R. L. and Seed, R. F. (1970). *British Journal of Anaesthesia*, **42**, 702.

Paton, W. D. M. and Zaimis, E. J. (1951). *Journal of Physiology, London*, **112**, 311.

Polstorff, K. and Schirmer, P. (1886). *Chemische Berichte*, **19**, 78.

Quevauviller, A. and Lainé, F. (1960). *Annales Pharmaceutiques Françaises*, **18**, 678.

Roquet, F., Harring, J., Godard, F. and Aurousseau, M. (1971). Communication to the European Medicinal Chemistry Congress at Lyon.

Saini, R. K. and Sharma, P. L. (1971). *Indian Journal of Medical Research*, **59**, 1104.

Savage, D. S., Cameron, A. F., Ferguson, G., Hannaway, C. and Mackay, I. R. (1971). *Journal of the Chemical Society B*, 410.

Saxena, P. R. and Bonta, I. L. (1970). *European Journal of Pharmacology*, **11**, 332.

Sellick, B. A. (1968). *Medical Annual*, 106.

Sharma, P. L. (1970). *Indian Journal of Medical Research*, **58**, 1736.

Singh, H., Paul, D. and Parashar, V. V. (1972). Abstracts IUPAC Symposium on the Chemistry of Natural Products, New Delhi, p. 247.

Smith, G., Proctor, D. W. and Spence, A. A. (1970). *British Journal of Anaesthesia*, **42**, 923.

Sohn, Y. J. and Aldrete, J. A. (1971). *Federation Proceedings*, **30**, 557.

Speight, T. M. and Avery, G. S. (1972). *Drugs*, **4**, 163.

Spiers, I. and Sim, A. W. (1972). *British Journal of Anaesthesia*, **44**, 370.

Standaert, F. G. (1964). *Journal of Pharmacology and Experimental Therapeutics*, **143**, 181.

Stephenson, R. P. (1948). *British Journal of Pharmacology and Chemotherapy*, **3**, 237.

Stovner, J. and Lund, I. (1970). *British Journal of Anaesthesia*, **42**, 953.

Stovner, J., Theodorsen, L. and Bjelke, E. (1971). *British Journal of Anaesthesia*, **43**, 953.

Strunin, L., Strunin, J. M., Layton, J., Sim, A. W. and Simpson, B. R. (1972). *British Journal of Anaesthesia*, **44**, 624.

Sugrue, M. F. and Duff, N. (1973). *Naunyn-Schmiedebergs Archives of Pharmacology*, **279**, Supplement Abstract, 48.

Sutor, D. J. (1963). *Journal of the Chemical Society*, 1105.

Veen, F. van der (1971). Unpublished data.

Verner, I. R. (1963). Communication to Royal Society of Medicine, London, April 5.

Visser, J. and Vies, J. van der (1968). Personal communication.

Waser, P. G. (1973). *Naunyn-Schmiedeberg's Archives of Pharmacology*, **279**, 399.

Wieriks, J. (1969). Proceedings of the Fourth International Symposium on Anaesthesia, Varna, p. 793.

Mechanisms in Angina Pectoris in Relation to Drug Therapy

BRIAN F. ROBINSON, MD, FRCP

St. George's Hospital, Hyde Park Corner, London, England

1 Introduction and history

Angina pectoris was first clearly described by Heberden in 1772, but it was not until the early 1930s that the cause of the symptom was finally agreed. It is now accepted that angina arises when the blood supply to some part of the myocardium has become inadequate for its metabolic needs. In the majority of patients who present with angina pectoris, the inadequacy of the myocardial blood supply results solely from the presence of atheromatous obstructions in the coronary arteries, and this discussion will not concern itself with the other factors, such as aortic valve disease and anaemia, which occasionally contribute to production of the symptom.

The first effective drug for the symptomatic relief of angina pectoris was amyl nitrite, introduced in 1867 by Lauder Brunton. He tried this drug because he thought that a rise in blood pressure was an important factor in precipitating pain and he reasoned that a reduction in pressure induced by a nitrite might be helpful in ending the attack. Amyl nitrite was found to be highly effective in relieving pain and the more convenient glyceryl trinitrate continues to be one of the most useful drugs in the management of angina. With the gradual recognition of the importance of coronary artery disease in the causation of pain, Brunton's original view that the nitrites worked by reducing the blood pressure (and hence the work of the heart) was abandoned and it became generally believed that they worked by dilating the coronary arteries. The model of angina that, consciously or unconsciously, had come to be accepted was one in which coronary flow was regarded as the dominant variable and changes in the work of the heart were thought of as only of secondary importance. The search for drugs which could be used in the symptomatic treatment of angina concentrated entirely on looking for substances which would be powerful coronary dilators. This effort led to the discovery of many coronary dilators, but few were effective in the treatment of angina. It is now realized that those "coronary dilators" that do have some therapeutic value almost certainly work by mechanisms other than their effect on the coronary arteries. There is little evidence that coronary flow can be increased at rest by ordinary doses of dilator drugs *in patients with diseased coronary arteries* and no evidence at all that the maximum response to raised metabolic demand can be increased. A minor contribution from redistribution of the available blood towards the areas of poor perfusion cannot be ruled out. It seems unlikely, however, that any action on the coronary circulation is of significant benefit since it has been shown that intra-coronary nitroglycerin is not effective in relieving angina provoked by pacing whereas systemic nitroglycerin will abolish pain (Ganz and Marcus, 1972). It is now apparent that the major action of all drugs which can be shown to be effective in the prevention or relief of anginal pain is a reduction in cardiac work rather than an increase in coronary flow. There can be few better examples of how the unwitting adoption of an incorrect model of drug action can lead to a vast amount of fruitless effort in the search for new drugs.

The model of angina which has evolved over the past ten years is one in which maximum coronary flow is taken to be relatively fixed and the work and metabolic requirements of the left ventricle are regarded as the major variable. The remainder of this discussion will be devoted to an analysis of the mechanisms by which the work of the left ventricle is determined and which are responsible for the precipitation of a critical degree of local myocardial ischaemia and so inducing an anginal attack.

2   Mechanisms determining onset of angina pectoris

2.1   DETERMINANTS OF LEFT VENTRICULAR OXYGEN REQUIREMENTS AND RELATION TO PRECIPITATION OF ANGINA

The main factors determining the work and oxygen requirements of the left ventricle are the heart rate, the tension developed in the myocardium and the myocardial contractility. The tension developed in the wall is a function of both systolic pressure and the radius of curvature, i.e. the ventricular dimensions. During repeated episodes of exercise or emotional stress under similar conditions, ventricular dimensions and contractility probably vary relatively little, and heart rate and systolic pressure become the major variables determining changes in left ventricular oxygen demands. In these circumstances, the product of heart rate and systolic pressure at the onset of anginal pain was found to be relatively constant in any one patient no matter what level of work was used to provoke the pain and the product was similar in a spontaneous attack at rest to that during exercise in the same patient (Robinson, 1967). A similar threshold for the production

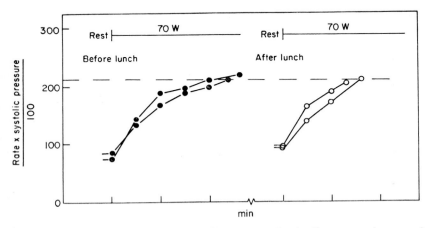

Fig. 1. Product of heart rate and systolic pressure in duplicate exercise tests in the same patient before and after lunch. Each test was terminated at the onset of angina. Exercise tolerance is reduced from about $2\frac{1}{2}$ minutes before lunch to $1\frac{1}{2}$ minutes after. This can be accounted for by the more rapid increase in rate–pressure product after eating.

of pain can be demonstrated in most patients when angina is provoked by cardiac pacing (Sowton *et al.*, 1967). It thus appears that each patient has a critical level for the work and oxygen requirements of the left ventricle at which pain can be expected to develop. Variations in the ease with which pain is provoked on different occasions almost certainly result from variations in the circulatory response to stress, although there is little direct evidence of this. It is known, however, that exposure to cold or a recent meal increases the circulatory response to a standard work load and both circumstances are well recognized as factors which favour the precipitation of angina. In a patient with angina studied before and after lunch, deterioration in exercise tolerance could be fully accounted for by increased circulatory response (Fig. 1).

2.2   MECHANISMS CONTROLLING LEFT VENTRICULAR OXYGEN REQUIREMENTS

How, then, are the determinants of left ventricular work controlled? *Heart rate* is controlled by the autonomic nervous system; the increase with exercise will not, however, be the same for any given work load on each occasion, but will vary depending on such factors as the level of physical training, emotional state, environmental conditions and the nature of the exercise. *Systolic pressure* will depend among other factors on cardiac output and peripheral arterial resistance. One of the major factors controlling cardiac output is the filling pressure; this will vary as a result of posture, but in any particular situation the most important controlling factor is variation in the degree of constriction in the systemic venous bed and this is under sympathetic control. Peripheral arterial resistance is, of course, also under the control of the sympathetic nervous system. The *size of the ventricle* is influenced by myocardial function and the filling pressure, both of which can be altered by the autonomic nervous system.

During exercise or emotional stress, there are thus four main ways in which the metabolic needs of the left ventricle can be influenced by the autonomic nervous system; they are changes in heart rate, changes in peripheral resistance, changes in the degree of venoconstriction, and changes in myocardial contractility. The quantitative importance of changes in contractility is less clear than that of the other three factors. With exercise, heart rate increases; peripheral resistance falls as a result of metabolic influences, but the fall is moderated by the constrictor influence of the sympathetic; the veins constrict; myocardial contractility is increased. When the work of the left ventricle has increased to a critical level which depends on the severity of the coronary artery disease, angina develops.

3   Circulatory changes induced by the anginal attack

Once ischaemia has been induced, there is evidence that this may itself induce circulatory changes which will tend to maintain or even increase myocardial work so that the anginal attack persists and may even get worse after the initiating stimulus has been withdrawn. The changes observed include an increase in the constriction of the veins and a rise in peripheral resistance with resultant increase in systolic pressure.

In normal subjects, the constriction of the veins provoked by exercise begins to wear off within 10–20 seconds of ceasing exertion. In 8 patients with angina in whom forearm venoconstriction could be demonstrated during exercise, 5 were observed to show an increase in constriction on at least one occasion during the anginal episode that was induced (Robinson *et al.*, 1970). It is not clear how this response is mediated, and it might merely be a response to pain. In a patient whose hand vein tone was followed continuously, however, abnormal and severe venoconstriction began to develop about 30 seconds before the subject was aware of pain which suggests the response may be triggered by the ischaemic episode and is not merely emotional in origin.

The abnormal response in the arterial system is manifest by changes in arterial pressure. In normal subjects, arterial pressure rises with exertion, but returns to resting levels with little delay when exercise is stopped. In a study in which 14 patients with angina pectoris performed repeated bouts of exercise on a bicycle ergometer, systolic pressure fell unduly slowly after at least one bout of exercise in 9 patients and in 4 patients the pressure was found to be *higher* after one minute of rest than it had been during exercise on at least one occasion (Robinson *et al.*, 1970). In a further patient who developed a prolonged episode of angina after exercise, this was associated with a rise in systolic pressure amounting to about 30 mmHg over the exercising level. An increase in pressure with rest is most unlikely to be caused by a rise in cardiac output, and it seems probable that it reflects an increase in peripheral resistance. As with the abnormal venous response, it is possible that the arterial response is initiated in some way by the onset of myocardial ischaemia. Whatever the mechanism of the venous and arterial responses, however, it is clear that they will tend to maintain and possibly even increase the load on the myocardium after the stress has stopped and in this way will tend to prolong the episode of pain. These mechanisms may account for the fact that angina is not always rapidly relieved by rest and that attacks once started may increase in severity despite removal of the precipitating stress. Harmful feedback mechanisms of this sort often provide fruitful opportunities in therapeutics if ways can be found of interrupting the loop at some point. There are, of course, many drugs available which will prevent arterial and venous constriction by interfering with the function of the sympathetic efferents or α-adreno-tropic receptors. Unfortunately, however, drugs acting in this way will only prevent unwanted reflex constriction at the expense of inhibiting the normal postural reflexes and so producing disabling postural hypotension. Some more specific way of preventing the unwanted reflex responses, possibly involving centrally acting drugs, will have to be found if this approach is to be made clinically useful.

4 Changes in myocardial blood flow

We have been thinking of coronary flow as essentially fixed, and, provided there are no major changes in aortic pressure, this assumption is probably true for total flow. Evidence is accumulating, however, that important changes may occur in local flow when angina is provoked. Maseri *et al.*

(1971) have studied local myocardial blood flow by following washout of a radioactive inert gas by means of a gamma camera. He has shown that blood flow in the centre of an ischaemic area may be much reduced during the anginal attack. The mechanisms involved in this severe disturbance of local blood flow are uncertain. One possibility is the occurrence of what we may call "coronary steal". If there are multiple obstructions in the coronary tree, a fall in resistance as a result of increased metabolic demand could increase flow through proximal branches with a resultant fall in flow

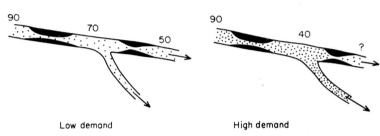

FIG. 2. Effect of increased metabolic demand on coronary flow when there are multiple stenoses. The fall in peripheral resistance would increase flow through the side branch with a resultant fall in flow through the stenotic distal vessel. The numerals indicate possible mean pressures in mmHg.

through more distal vessels (Fig. 2). It seems unlikely that any pharmacological method could be found to overcome this. Another factor which may influence local flow is the diastolic pressure in the left ventricle. If, as a result of proximal obstructions, the perfusion pressure is low in the smaller coronary arteries, a rise in diastolic pressure in the ventricle could reduce transmural pressure in vessels supplying the inner part of the heart muscle to such an extent that flow was brought to a halt. Large rises in ventricular diastolic pressure have been observed with the onset of anginal attacks (O'Brien et al., 1969; Parker et al., 1969), so we have here yet another mechanism by which angina, once initiated, may set up a self-perpetuating cycle.

5   Model for the circulatory changes in angina related to the action of drugs

There thus appears to be a complex interrelating series of mechanisms which may play a part in the initiation and maintenance of the myocardial ischaemia which is the cause of anginal pain. One possible model is shown in Fig. 3.

It is of some interest to see how existing anti-anginal drugs might be working in a model such as this. Glyceryl trinitrate lowers arterial pressure and so reduces the work of the left ventricle. This is achieved in part by its effect on the arterial system; it may also result from reduced cardiac output, however, and this is the consequence of the powerful dilator action of the nitrates on the venous system which leads to a reduction in both

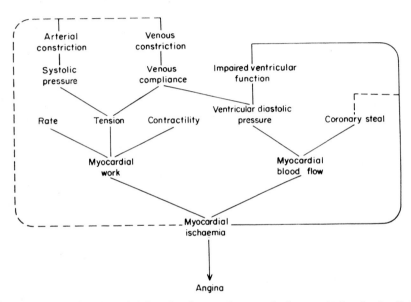

FIG. 3. Hypothetical model for circulatory changes during anginal episode. Solid lines indicate relationships that are well established. Interrupted lines show relationships for which there is evidence, but which are less certainly established.

cardiac filling pressure and ventricular size (Williams *et al.*, 1965). Glyceryl trinitrate thus reduces the work of the left ventricle in two ways: it lowers systolic pressure and it also reduces ventricular size. In addition to this action on ventricular work, it could theoretically prevent diversion of coronary flow from the inner layers of the myocardium by averting excessive rises in left ventricular diastolic pressure. Possibly it is this combination of beneficial effects that makes the short-acting organic nitrates so effective in the symptomatic management of angina pectoris. On the debit side, however, glyceryl trinitrate increases heart rate as a reflex result of the fall in blood pressure and this will increase cardiac work.

The β-blockers, and other drugs, such as prenylamine, which reduce sympathetic stimulation of the heart, will moderate the rise in heart rate with exercise and will also tend to reduce arterial pressure and contractility. Increased exercise tolerance after these drugs can always be accounted for by the reduction in heart rate (Robinson, 1971). Patients rarely achieve all the benefit expected from the lower heart rate, however, and they commonly develop pain after the drug at a lower heart rate than before, albeit at a higher level of external work. There is evidence that β-blockers increase ventricular size (Chamberlain, 1966), and it may be that this action offsets their beneficial effects to a greater or lesser extent.

Glyceryl trinitrate would be expected to reduce any increase in heart size after a β-blocker, while a β-blocker will reduce the increase in heart rate after organic nitrates. It is thus not surprising that the two groups of drugs may act synergistically, and it does not seem necessary to invoke effects on the coronary circulation to explain this.

There will almost certainly be mechanisms involved in the anginal episode which have not been considered in this model. It is suggested, however, that it provides a useful way of thinking about the action of drugs in angina pectoris and may provide insight into important aspects of the action of existing drugs. Better understanding of the mechanisms by which drugs of known efficacy exert their beneficial effects in angina would provide a rational starting point for the development of new therapeutic substances.

References

Chamberlain, D. A. (1966). *American Journal of Cardiology*, **18**, 321.

Ganz, W. and Marcus, H. S. (1972). *Circulation*, **46**, 880.

Maseri, di A., Mangini, P., L'Abbate, A., Pesola, A. and Conti, C. (1971). *Bollettino della Società Italiana di Cardiologia*, **16**, 531.

O'Brien, K. P., Higgs, L. M., Glancy, D. L. and Epstein, S. E. (1969). *Circulation*, **39**, 735.

Parker, J. O., Ledwich, J. R., West, R. O. and Case, R. B. (1969). *Circulation*, **39**, 745.

Robinson, B. F. (1967). *Circulation*, **35**, 1073.

Robinson, B. F., Collier, J., Nachev, Ch. and Wilson, A. G. (1970). *In* "Coronary Heart Disease and Physical Fitness" (Eds O. A. Larsen and R. O. Malmborg). Munksgaard, Copenhagen.

Robinson, B. F. (1971). *Postgraduate Medical Journal*, **47**, suppl. 41.

Sowton, G. E., Balcon, R., Cross, D. and Frick, M. H. (1967). *Cardiovascular Research*, **1**, 301.

Williams, J. F., Glick, G. and Braunwald, E. (1965). *Circulation*, **32**, 767.

Interferon and Interferon Inducers

D. H. METZ, MSc, PhD

National Institute for Medical Research, Mill Hill, London, England

1   Introduction

1.1   BACKGROUND

The phenomenon of viral interference has been known for many years. This term is used to describe the situation when the presence of one virus interferes with the replication of another in some particular cell culture or animal. It was while studying this effect in chick chorioallantoic membranes infected with influenza virus that Isaacs and Lindenmann (1957) discovered interferon. Most though not all examples of viral interference are mediated by interferon.

The interferon system is a normal defensive response of an animal to virus infection. The essence of the phenomenon is as follows: (1) virus infection of animal cells results in the synthesis and release of interferon which is a cellular protein; (2) when uninfected cells come into contact with interferon they become resistant to subsequent infection by viruses.

The outstanding interest of the interferon mechanism lies in the fact that it is not specific for a particular virus. All animal viruses induce interferon synthesis to a greater or lesser extent and the replication of all such viruses in interferon-treated cells is inhibited, again to a greater or lesser extent.

The following criteria serve to distinguish interferon from other less specific inhibitors (Lockart, 1973). First, interferon is active against a wide range of unrelated viruses. Second, interferon is usually cell specific; that is to say it is active on homologous cells and not on heterologous cells. For example, interferon made in human cells is not active on mouse cells and vice versa. Interferons are not tissue specific. Third, interferon is not toxic to cells. Fourth, interferon is not directly antiviral but acts through an intracellular effect which requires functional host cell metabolism. Fifth, interferons are proteins which are usually stable at pH 2. This brief outline should serve to orient the reader to what follows.

Obviously questions both of a fundamental and of a practical nature are suggested by the interferon phenomenon as described above. Among the more important are the mechanism by which a virus induces the synthesis of interferon, the nature of the substance itself, the mechanism by which it renders a cell resistant to infection, and the possibilities for the therapy of virus diseases. These topics form the subject matter of the sections of this review that follow. The emphasis will be both on those aspects of the subject which seem most securely extablished and on the biochemical mechanisms involved. References will be selective rather than comprehensive. Commonly, citations will be to recent references or reviews which should serve as an entry into the literature of the particular topic. For more detailed general accounts of interferon the reader is referred to the concise monograph by Vilček (1969) and the comprehensive multi-author volume edited by Finter (1973a). Other useful recent reviews include those of Colby (1971), Colby and Morgan (1971), Ng and Vilček (1972) and Kleinschmidt (1972).

1.2 ASSAY OF INTERFERON

The only way to detect interferon is to measure its ability to inhibit virus replication. Estimation of interferon therefore involves a biological assay with all the variability that this implies. Perhaps the most commonly used is the plaque reduction assay. Typically, monolayers of suitable cells are treated with a range of dilutions of the interferon preparation and are incubated at 37°C for 4–18 hours. The interferon is then removed and about 50–80 plaque-forming units of a suitably sensitive virus are inoculated onto each dish. After a period of absorption of the virus (1–2 hours usually) the monolayers are overlaid with nutrient agar and are incubated for a sufficient time for plaques to appear. The dishes are stained and the plaques counted. The titre of the interferon preparation is usually defined as the reciprocal of the dilution which decreases the number of plaques per dish by 50 per cent. Other modes of interferon assay that are frequently used include the reduction of virus yield in a single cycle growth and inhibition of a virus-induced cytopathic effect. The subject of interferon assay has been recently reviewed by Finter (1973b).

The dose–response relationships in these assays are sigmoidal curves with an approximately linear portion between 20 and 80 per cent of the response. Dose–response curves for different interferon preparations assayed in the same system should be parallel.

Both viruses and cells vary in their sensitivity to interferon and it is usually desirable to choose a virus–cell combination that displays an optimal response. Clearly the titre of an interferon preparation will depend on the assay system used. In order to be able to make comparisons between different laboratories there are now available reference preparations each containing an arbitrary but defined number of "reference units" per ampoule (Finter, 1973b). It is desirable that published data should be expressed in these units or at least in a manner that can be related to them.

2 The Synthesis of interferon

2.1 INTERFERON INDUCTION BY VIRUSES AND BY NONVIRAL SUBSTANCES

Viruses and a variety of nonviral substances, particularly natural and synthetic polyanions, will induce the synthesis of interferon when introduced into cell cultures or animals. Representatives of all major groups of viruses have been shown to induce interferon synthesis (Ho, 1973a). Myxoviruses and arboviruses are the two groups that have been most widely used and are the most effective inducers. Interferon may be produced when live virus infects permissible cells so that progeny virus is made. It may also be produced when certain inactivated viruses are employed, for example ultraviolet inactivated myxoviruses, or when nonpermissive cells, in which the virus does not grow, are infected with certain types of live virus. Thus virus replication is not essential for interferon synthesis. While it is apparent that viruses vary rather widely in their interferon inducing ability the reasons for this are poorly understood. One factor, doubtless, is the ability of the virus to switch off cellular macromolecular synthesis; viruses, such as the picornaviruses, which are efficient in this respect, tend to be poor inducers.

The most significant class of nonviral inducers of interferon are the synthetic double-stranded polynucleotides. Hilleman and his colleagues at the Merck Institute first demonstrated that the active component of helenine, a substance extracted from *Penicillium funiculosum* which was known to induce interferon synthesis, was a double-stranded RNA species (Lampson *et al.*, 1967). They subsequently found that a wide variety of double-stranded polynucleotides from natural and synthetic sources were active inducers (Field *et al.*, 1967a, 1967b; Tytell *et al.*, 1967). These initial observations stimulated a great deal of industry in many laboratories from which the following conclusions may be drawn (for a more extensive discussion, see the reviews of Colby, 1971 and Colby and Morgan, 1971). Double-stranded polynucleotides are interferon inducers in cell culture and in animals. In culture the effect may be studied either by measuring interferon synthesis or by observing the development of resistance of the cells to subsequent virus infection. Commonly, detection of interferon synthesis requires substantially higher doses (by a factor of about 10^4) of the polynucleotide than does detection of resistance to virus infection. Resistance to infection is found with doses as low as $0 \cdot 000\ 004$ μg ml^{-1} which is equivalent to about two polynucleotide molecules per cell (De Clercq *et al.*, 1971). Clearly double-stranded polynucleotides are very potent substances. Although they are known to give rise to a variety of phenomena when applied to cells or animals other than interferon induction (Beers and Braun, 1971; Talal, 1971), it seems likely, on balance, that the induction of resistance to virus infection is mediated by the interferon mechanism, even at doses when interferon synthesis cannot be detected. One item of evidence in support of this view is the finding that virus replication in a line of cells which was able to respond to interferon but was unable to make it was not inhibited by treatment with double-stranded polyinosinic-polycytidylic acid, (poly(I).poly(C)) (Schafer and Lockart, 1970).

The helical, base-paired, double-stranded secondary structure of the polynucleotide is important for interferon induction. There is evidence, however, that some single-stranded polynucleotides are able to induce cellular resistance to viral infection but this only occurs at doses 1000-fold greater than that at which the double-stranded polymers are effective (Baron *et al.*, 1969; De Clercq and Merigan, 1969). It is possible that this is due to the presence of secondary structure which is known to occur in some single-stranded polynucleotides. Triple-stranded, helical polynucleotides, however, are inactive as inducers (De Clercq *et al.*, 1974).

While double-stranded RNA is a good inducer of interferon, double-stranded DNA is not (Lampson *et al.*, 1967). DNA and double-stranded polydeoxyribonucleotides have been found to be inactive as inducers (Colby and Chamberlin, 1969) or only active at rather high concentrations (100 to 10 000-fold greater than for polyribonucleotides; De Clercq *et al.*,

1970). Furthermore, double-stranded structures in which one strand is a polyribonucleotide and the other is a polydeoxyribonucleotide are inactive, except perhaps at high doses, and this is not due to the failure of these hybrid polymers to be taken up into the cell or to enhanced intracellular breakdown (Colby and Chamberlin, 1969). It appears, therefore, that for a double-stranded polynucleotide to be an effective interferon inducer at low concentrations both 2'-hydroxyls on the sugar moieties must be free. Confirmation of this view is provided by the finding that replacement of the 2'-hydroxyl group by a variety of substituents markedly diminishes the interferon inducing ability (Black et al., 1972; De Clercq et al., 1972b; De Clercq and Janik, 1973; Torrence et al., 1973). Replacement of the purine N-7 atom by carbon also abolishes interferon inducing ability (De Clercq et al., 1974).

In contrast to the rather stringent requirement for secondary structure, it appears that no particular sequence of bases (primary structure) is necessary for interferon-inducing ability. Not only are naturally occurring double-stranded RNAs from a wide variety of sources very efficient inducers but the associated homopolymers poly(I).poly(C) are as effective as the alternating copolymer poly(I-C) (Colby and Chamberlin, 1969).

Within the class of double-stranded, polyribonucleotides, interferon inducing ability can vary over a wide range (De Clercq et al., 1970; Colby, 1971). The minimum concentration of polymer in cell culture required to render the cells resistant to infection may vary between 0·000 004 and 1 μg ml^{-1}, depending on the chemical composition, and the conditions used. In decreasing order of efficiency we have poly(I).poly(C), poly(I-C), poly(G).poly(C), poly(I).poly(BrC), poly(A-U), poly(A-BrU), poly-(A).poly(U). While we do not fully understand the reason for this variation in interferon inducing ability with base composition, a number of factors doubtless contribute and these will now be considered.

The melting temperature (T_m; the temperature at which the double-helical structure is disrupted into the two constituent strands) is generally supposed to be a relevant factor in view of the requirement for secondary structure. The results of Colby and Chamberlin (1969) and of De Clercq and Merigan (1969) suggested that antiviral activity increased with thermal stability in the range 40°C to 60°C while above 60°C there was no correlation between activity and melting temperature. The sensitivity of the poly-nucleotide to ribonuclease present in the cells or in the surrounding medium is a factor that might be expected to be important. Certainly, when the phosphate group of poly(A-U) was replaced by a thiophosphate the resulting polymer was 10 to 100 times more resistant to pancreatic ribonuclease and was 100 to 10 000 times more active in inducing cellular resistance (De Clercq et al., 1969). This modification had no effect on the thermal stability. On the other hand, an absence of correlation between ribonuclease resistance and antiviral effect has been found for a number of other poly-nucleotides (Colby and Chamberlin, 1969). There is some evidence supporting an inverse relationship between the inability of different cultured cell types to degrade poly(I).poly(C) and the level of interferon produced in the cells (De Clercq and Stewart, 1974).

The molecular weight of the component strands may affect the antiviral activity of the double-helical polynucleotide. Although the data are to some extent conflicting, it appears in general that the antiviral activity decreases as the size of either strand decreases (Niblack and McCreary, 1971). Decreasing the size of the poly(I) strand of poly(I).poly(C) reduces interferon induction to a greater extent than does reducing the size of the poly(C) strand (Stewart and De Clercq, 1974). Nevertheless, a complex between poly(C) and an oligo(I) six nucleotides in length still has significant antiviral activity (Pitha and Carter, 1971a).

The first step in interferon induction by double-stranded polynucleotides appears to be rapid binding to the cell surface which can occur either at 4°C or 37°C (Bausek and Merigan, 1969). It might be supposed that the chemical composition of the polynucleotide may affect the rate and persistence of binding. A thorough study failed to demonstrate a correlation between either of these factors and the antiviral effect for a number of poly-nucleotides (De Clercq et al., 1972a). This presumably means that variation in binding was not the limiting factor in the development of the antiviral effect in the examples studied. In addition to the binding of the poly-nucleotide to the surface of the cell, binding to an intracellular receptor may be necessary and different chemical species might also differ in their efficiency in this respect. There is evidence that poly(I).poly(C) linked to a solid support is as active an inducer as the free polynucleotide (Pitha and Pitha, 1973; Taylor-Papadimitriou and Kallos, 1973). This would imply that the inducer does not need to enter the cell and hence that the receptor must be on the cell surface. These experiments are not entirely conclusive, however, since a small amount of the polynucleotide is released from the support while it is in contact with the cells.

The ability of a given polynucleotide such as poly(I).poly(C) to induce interferon synthesis or cellular resistance to infection varies according to the type of cell used. It has been found that when only a small effect is obtained the addition of a polycation such as diethylaminoethyl-dextran (DEAE-dextran) or polylysine often results in considerable enhancement (Dianzani et al., 1968). Such polycations may facilitate uptake of the polynucleotide and perhaps protect it from enzymic degradation (Bausek and Merigan, 1969; Pitha and Carter, 1971b; Wacker et al., 1972). Little is known, however, of the nature of the interaction between polynucleotide and polycations and hence other mechanisms for facilitation cannot be excluded (Carter *et al.*, 1972). A number of double-stranded polynucleotides, in particular the alternating copolymer poly(A-U), may be thermally activated by incubation at 37°C prior to their coming into contact with cells. Increases in antiviral activity of up to 10^6-fold have been reported (De Clercq *et al.*, 1971). The mechanism of this effect is unclear although it may involve slippage of a branched helical structure to a longer unbranched structure. Sequential administration of the complementary polynucleotides poly(I) and poly(C) to cell cultures may result in a greater antiviral activity than that resulting from addition of the preformed double-stranded complex (De Clercq and De Somer, 1972). It is thought that the two strands probably recombine at the cell membrane.

While all the factors discussed above probably affect the efficacy of a polynucleotide as an interferon inducer the available data do not permit a definitive statement concerning their relative importance. Indeed, this may well depend on the test system employed. It is known, for example, that levels of serum ribonuclease vary between different animal species and this may limit the ability of a double-stranded polynucleotide to induce interferon *in vivo*. Nevertheless, it does appear that there are definite minimum values for the thermal stability, nuclease resistance and chain length below which interferon induction is not observed; in an intermediate range interferon inducing ability is proportional to the thermal stability, etc., while increase above a maximum value leads to no additional enhancement of induction.

Viruses and double-stranded polynucleotides induce interferon synthesis both in cell culture and in animals. There are a variety of other organisms and substances which in general induce interferon synthesis in animals only, often requiring intravenous or intraperitoneal injection of relatively large doses (see De Clercq and Merigan, 1970; Colby and Morgan, 1971; and Merigan, 1973a, for complete listings). Presumably the reason for the absence of activity in cell cultures is that the cells which respond to these inducers do not attach to glass or plastic and hence are not readily cultured. There is some evidence, however, that many of these inducers act only on cells of the lymphoreticular system, which is responsible for the organism's immune response (Ng and Vilček, 1972).

Apart from the viruses, a variety of other microorganisms induce interferon synthesis. These include bacteria, protozoa, rickettsiae and chlamydia. Many of these are intracellular parasites and conceivably partially double-stranded RNA of the organism is thereby introduced into the cell. Various microbial extracts induce interferon and two of them are of particular interest. Extracts from a variety of Penicillium strains have antiviral and interferon-inducing activity. The antiviral activity of a *P. funiculosum* filtrate was first demonstrated in 1948 (Shope, 1948). It was later found that a similar extract from *P. stoloniferum* (known as statolon) would induce interferon synthesis and the active principle was thought to be a complex anionic polysaccharide (Kleinschmidt *et al.*, 1964). It turned out, however, that the active principle was in fact a fungal virus (Kleinschmidt and Ellis, 1967) which, as noted earlier for the similar case of helenine, contained double-stranded RNA. It is possible that the interferon inducing ability of other microorganisms may be due to their harbouring double-stranded RNA viruses. Statolon and similar fungal extracts are, as one would expect, active in cell culture as well as in the animal.

The other interesting class of materials extracted from microorganisms that induce interferon synthesis in animals are bacterial lipopolysaccharides (e.g. endotoxins). In the case of the material from *Salmonella typhimurium* it appears that it is the fatty acid moiety that is responsible for the effect (Younger *et al.*, 1973). This material does not appear to contain any RNA. It is likely that the activity of those Gram-negative bacteria which induce interferon synthesis in animals is due to endotoxin.

Another class of inducers of interferon which clearly lack RNA content are the synthetic polymers. These consist of a variety of anionic polymers and copolymers including polyacrylic and polymethacrylic acids, maleic anhydride copolymers and polyvinyl sulphate (Merigan, 1973a). The requirements for interferon-inducing ability are a stable long-chain backbone on which negatively charged groups are placed in a regular and dense sequence.

The final class of inducers to be considered are the recently discovered class of low molecular weight inducers, typified by tilorone hydrochloride (**1**) (Mayer and Krueger, 1970). This drug, which is the water-soluble dihydrochloride salt of 2,7-bis(2-diethylaminoethoxy)fluoren-9-one, has a broad spectrum of antiviral activity when given orally to mice and acts by inducing interferon synthesis. It does not, however, induce interferon in a variety of mouse cell cultures (De Clercq and Merigan, 1971). Another low

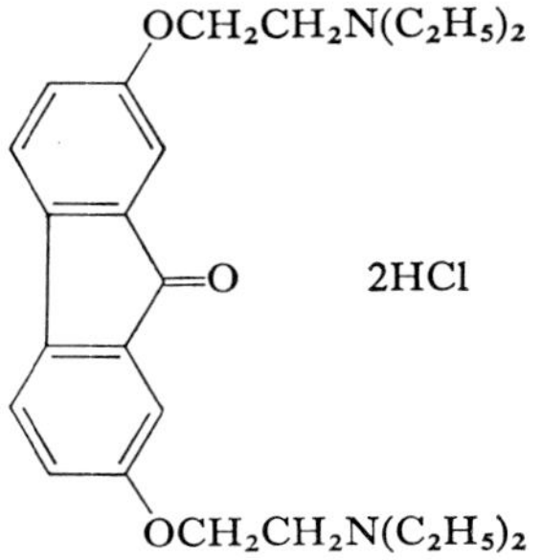

$OCH_2CH_2N(C_2H_5)_2$

$=O$ 2HCl

$OCH_2CH_2N(C_2H_5)_2$

(**1**)

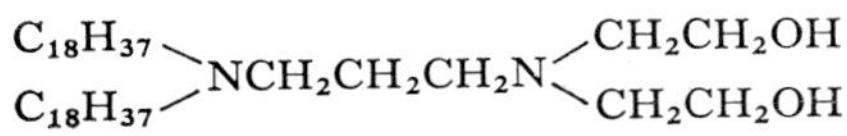

$$C_{18}H_{37} \diagdown NCH_2CH_2CH_2N \diagup ^{CH_2CH_2OH}_{CH_2CH_2OH}$$
$$C_{18}H_{37} \diagup$$

(**2**)

molecular weight inducer is NN-dioctadecyl-$N'N'$-bis(2-hydroxyethyl)-propanediamine (2); this is active when injected into mice though not when administered orally (Hoffman *et al.*, 1973).

In concluding this section on interferon inducers it should be observed that all inducers are, to a greater or lesser extent, toxic to cells and animals (Stinebring and Absher, 1971; Black *et al.*, 1973). As we shall discuss later (section 5.2) this is an important factor when one considers the practicality of the use of interferon inducers for therapy or prophylaxis.

2.2   CELLULAR FACTORS IN INTERFERON SYNTHESIS

The role of the cell is just as important as that of the viral or nonviral inducer in the synthesis of interferon. Cells from many mammalian and avian species have been demonstrated to make interferon as have cells from at least one species of reptile and of fish (Vilček, 1969; Ho, 1973b). While cell cultures vary markedly in their ability to make interferon in response to a given inducer it does not seem possible to make any useful generalization from the available data. It should be stressed that it is the interaction of inducer and cell that determines the extent of interferon production and not the intrinsic capability of the inducer or the cell alone. Thus, for example, Newcastle disease virus (NDV) is a poor inducer in chick embryo cells but a good inducer in mouse L cells while other viruses, such as the arboviruses, are good inducers in chick cells.

Primary cultures usually contain a heterogeneous population of cell types with different morphological and physiological properties and these may respond differently to inducers. There is good evidence that in primary cultures of mouse kidney cells there exist functionally two types of cell, each of which responds to only one of the pair of inducers, NDV and poly(I).poly(C) (Stewart *et al.*, 1971a). It is known also that different sublines of cells that originally derived from one culture may have different capacities to produce interferon (Cantell and Paucker, 1963). For practical purposes it is obviously desirable to select cell lines which yield high titres of interferon. The recent finding of a line of transformed mouse cells which produced as much as 100 000 units per ml in response to NDV, this being about 100-fold more than was produced in the more commonly used mouse L cells, is an interesting example of what can be achieved in this direction (Oie *et al.*, 1972).

Interferon synthesis in intact animals is very dependent on the species employed. Mice and some other rodents respond to intravenous inoculation with large doses of a variety of viruses by synthesizing sizeable quantities of interferon which is detectable in the serum (Baron and Buckler, 1963). But in other species, such as man, only low serum interferon titres are found. The serum interferon levels found in different strains of inbred mice in response to a given dose of inducer may vary significantly; thus the mean titres for NDV-induced serum interferon differed by a factor of six when the Balb/c and C_{57} Black strains were compared (De Maeyer and De Maeyer-Guignard, 1969). In this example, a genetic analysis, which involved crossing the two strains, indicated that there was a single factor responsible for the difference in interferon production which was partly dominant and autosomal. It is interesting that the C_{57}Bl strain (the high producer) is known to be relatively resistant to virus infections. Recently, three more genetic loci have been identified which affect the interferon response to other viruses (E. De Maeyer, personal communication).

The question of which cells in the intact animal are the source of interferon is a difficult one to approach experimentally. In general it appears that the types of cells involved differs from one system to another and depends on numerous factors such as the type of inducer, the dose, the route of inoculation and the choice of animal. Available data suggest that interferon is commonly made at the site of maximum virus multiplication (Vilček, 1969). The early appearance of circulating interferon in animals inoculated intravenously with large doses of virus suggests that the cells responsible are easily accessible from the circulation. Cells of the reticulo-endothelial system are likely candidates in this respect. It has been found that relatively low doses of X-irradiation of mice would substantially reduce the amount of circulating interferon induced by four myxoviruses while interferon induction by encephalomyocarditis virus or vaccinia virus was very resistant to irradiation (De Maeyer et al., 1969). Induction by other viruses was of intermediate sensitivity. This suggested that a number of distinct cell populations were responsible for interferon synthesis, each responding to one or more different viruses. When irradiated mice were treated (grafted) with bone marrow cells from another animal of the same inbred strain interferon-producing capacity was restored. Furthermore, when irradiated mice received bone marrow cells from a rat, interferon-producing capacity was again restored but now the interferon had the species specificity of rat interferon (De Maeyer-Guignard et al., 1969). This demonstrated that the circulating interferon, at least in the case when NDV is the inducer, was made in bone marrow-derived cells.

In addition to those already discussed, a rather wide variety of factors are known to influence interferon synthesis in cell culture and in animals. These will be mentioned quite briefly since the underlying mechanisms are obscure. Fuller accounts are available (Vilček, 1969; Ho, 1973b). Interferon pretreatment of cells prior to induction affects subsequent interferon synthesis. This is known as "priming". Priming may enhance the amount of interferon produced, it may accelerate its timing, or it may inhibit interferon production. The extent of enhancement can be quite marked. Thus no interferon was made by mouse L cells when they were infected by MM virus but several thousand units were produced when the cells were pretreated with ten units prior to infection (Stewart *et al.*, 1971b). When priming enhances synthesis it might be supposed that this is due to the priming dose of interferon blocking some viral function that normally switches off interferon synthesis by the cell, and, conversely, when priming inhibits interferon production, the synthesis of some necessary viral component for induction might be blocked. Available evidence, however, indicates that this rationale is at the very least an oversimplification (Stewart *et al.*, 1971b) (see section 4.3).

Following interferon induction in cell culture or in animals, there frequently occurs a "refractory state". During the duration of this state further induction does not result in interferon production. In the case of L cells induced by NDV the refractoriness of the cells to further induction was lost by the time two cell divisions had occurred in a dividing culture but was not lost in the same period if the cells were kept in stationary phase (Paucker and Boxaca, 1967). The existence of the refractory state is of obvious importance when one comes to consider the practical use of interferon inducers in animals and man (section 5).

Other factors that have been reported to affect interferon production include the age of cells in culture or of animals, temperature, steroid hormones, stress, and carcinogens. Antimetabolites may inhibit interferon production and the effects of these will be considered in the following section on the mechanism of interferon synthesis.

A final point to be discussed in the present section is the question of "preformed interferon". Observations that the induction in mice by certain nonviral inducers such as endotoxin resulted in a more rapid release of interferon than did that by viral inducers, and that inhibitors of protein synthesis failed to block induction by the former class while markedly suppressing synthesis by the latter, lead to the suggestion that endotoxin stimulated the release of preformed interferon while viruses caused *de novo* synthesis (Younger *et al.*, 1965). The interpretation of the inhibitor experiments has been questioned, however, and other explanations are possible for the different kinetic behaviour, and so the question of the existence of preformed interferon in significant amounts in the animal is still open (Ng and Vilček, 1972).

2.3   MECHANISM OF INTERFERON SYNTHESIS

The production of interferon requires the *induction* step followed by *synthesis* and release of the interferon molecule. In this section we consider first the synthesis of interferon and then the mechanism of induction (Burke, 1973).

It is established that interferon is a protein (see section 3.2). Initial observations that interferon synthesis was induced by viruses implied that interferon could be either a cellular or a viral portein, the genetic information being coded either by the cellular DNA or by the viral nucleic acid. The fact that double-stranded polynucleotides are potent interferon inducers is a strong argument against virus coding. Another and earlier argument in this direction arose from the use of the antimetabolite actino-mycin D which inhibits RNA synthesis (transcription) from a DNA template. Thus, while the drug inhibits RNA synthesis directed by the cell and by DNA viruses, most RNA viruses, whose replication does not involve DNA, are not affected. It was therefore possible to demonstrate that actinomycin D could inhibit interferon synthesis without inhibiting replication of an RNA virus (Heller, 1963). This showed that cellular RNA synthesis was required for interferon synthesis and it is generally thought that the particular species is the messenger RNA for the interferon protein. The recent observation that an inhibitor with the characteristics of mouse interferon was produced by chick or monkey cells incubated with RNA extracted from interferon-producing mouse cells suggests how the pre-sumptive interferon messenger RNA may be further characterized (De Maeyer-Guignard et al., 1972; Montagnier et al., 1974). Studies in which actinomycin D was added at various times following addition of the inducer suggested that synthesis of the interferon messenger RNA is complete in 2–5 hours and that it is quite stable (Wagner, 1964; Vilček and Havell, 1973).

As interferon is a protein, protein synthesis inhibitors suppress its forma-tion (Wagner and Huang, 1965). If interferon is specified by a cellular gene then this may be expected to be located on a particular chromosome. Analy-sis of a number of mouse–monkey hybrid cell lines, only one of which pro-duced monkey interferon, indicated that this gene was probably located on a small subtelocentric chromosome (Cassingena et al., 1971). Similarly analy-sis of mouse–human hybrid cell lines showed that both human chromosomes 2 and 5 were required for interferon production (Tan et al., 1974).

Turning now to the mechanism of induction, we must consider both the cellular components that respond to the inducing entity and the nature of this entity itself. Very little information is available concerning the former. Nevertheless, various model mechanisms, taken from other systems, have been discussed in this context (Ng and Vilček, 1972).

By analogy with the model of Jacob and Monod (1961), designed to explain enzymic induction in bacterial systems, one can postulate the existence of a repressor molecule which acts to block the transcription of the messenger RNA for the interferon molecule. The inducer would bind to the repressor, thereby inactivating it, and thus the mRNA would be synthesized and then translated to yield interferon. An alternative model, also involving a repressor, may be derived from that of Tomkins *et al.* (1969) which was formulated to explain enzymic induction by steroid hormones in cultured liver cells. Here a labile repressor molecule binds to the mRNA thereby blocking translation. The inducer may either bind to the repressor to block its function, or it might act in some way to block its synthesis. Both of these models involve a repression of interferon synthesis. One might also consider models based on activation, perhaps by analogy with the bacterial sigma factor which stimulates the activity of RNA polymerase (Burgess *et al.*, 1969). Here, it might be supposed, the combination of a receptor molecule with the inducer would serve to activate transcription, or even translation, of the interferon messenger.

While all these models are plausible there is no available evidence which would permit us to discriminate between them. There is no direct evidence to support the existence of a repressor although there are results that have been taken to imply the existence of a cellular receptor for the inducer. The high potency of the double-stranded polynucleotide inducers coupled with the rather stringent structural requirements already discussed suggest that induction may involve a combination between a specific cellular receptor site and the inducer and that the extent of induction may be proportional to the amount of this complex formed. The molecular nature of the receptor would determine the range of structures permissible as inducers. Colby and Chamberlin (1969), who postulated the existence of such a receptor, also argued that it would probably be a protein since there are many examples of very specific protein–nucleic interactions, but all the specific nucleic acid–nucleic acid interactions known involve base-pairing interactions and, as noted previously, there is no evidence that the nucleotide sequence of the inducer is at all important.

It is, of course, an attractive hypothesis that double-stranded poly-ribonucleotides are the only high potency interferon inducers, and if this is indeed the case then it follows that viruses must act as inducers by synthesizing double-stranded RNA. We will consider the available evidence on just which presumably common components of the various viruses and of their replication cycles are responsible for interferon induction in the light of this hypothesis.

The replication of single-stranded RNA viruses involves a "replicative intermediate" which consists of a strand of viral RNA (the plus strand), a strand of RNA complementary to it (the minus strand), and the RNA polymerase enzyme. Synthesis of progeny plus strands involves the polymerase transcribing the minus strand. Although it is believed that the plus and minus strands do not for the most part form a regular double helix in the cell, it does appear that a certain amount of double-stranded RNA may accumulate especially at later times in infection (Baltimore, 1969). The RNA polymerase may prevent the formation of the double-stranded structure and loss of the enzyme from the replicating intermediate will presumably allow it to form. Thus the presence of this double-stranded viral RNA in cells infected with single-stranded RNA viruses may be sufficient to account for the induction of interferon by this class of viruses.

A study of interferon induction by temperature-sensitive mutants of Semliki forest virus, a single-stranded RNA virus (Lomniczi and Burke, 1970), has led to conclusions not inconsistent with this view. One class of such mutants are unable to synthesize viral RNA at 39°C (though they will do so at 30°C and hence may be grown at this temperature) and these will not induce interferon synthesis at 39°C, at least when a low multiplicity of infection (virus to cell ratio) is used. On the other hand both the wild-type virus and the class of mutants that will make viral RNA at the higher temperature, but which are defective in some later function, induce interferon synthesis at 39°C. These results indicate that viral RNA is needed for interferon induction. In addition it was observed at high multiplicities mutants which did not make RNA at 39°C would in fact induce interferon synthesis at this temperature. It has since been found, however, that unpurified stocks of a number of types of single-stranded RNA viruses may contain up to 2 per cent double-stranded RNA and this may well be the explanation for the apparently anomalous observation (Field *et al.*, 1972). Another study has employed temperature-sensitive mutants of Sindbis virus, a similar single-stranded RNA virus (Lockart *et al.*, 1968). Again, a mutant which did not make viral RNA at the higher temperature failed to induce interferon synthesis but a mutant which was able to make over 80 per cent of the normal amount of RNA induced only 10 per cent of the normal amount of interferon. This lack of quantitative correlation between RNA synthesis and interferon induction was also observed by Lomniczi and Burke (1970) who speculated that the conformation of the viral RNA synthesized in cells infected with the mutants was unfavourable for interferon formation. Alternatively, it may be that the amount of intracellular, double-stranded RNA formed may be less in the case of this particular group of mutants.

A recent study, emphasizing the difficulties of interpreting experiments using temperature-sensitive mutants, noted that the induction of interferon may occur at the restrictive temperature both through the reversion of the mutant to wild-type and through the leakiness of the mutant (Atkins *et al.*, 1974). The cautious conclusion was nevertheless drawn that a low threshold level of RNA synthesis is probably necessary for interferon induction by Sindbis virus.

A well-studied single-stranded RNA virus is Newcastle Disease virus (NDV), which is a good inducer of interferon in cultured cells of its natural host (chick embryo cells) only after ultraviolet irradiation. This virus has a virion RNA polymerase, i.e. this enzyme is an integral part of the virus. The irradiated virus retains the capacity to induce RNA synthesis both *in vitro* and in the infected cell, although with large doses of irradiation both the ability to synthesize RNA and to induce interferon are lost in parallel (Clavell and Bratt, 1971). The RNA made by the irradiated virus appears to have some double-stranded structure and is, therefore, a plausible candidate for the inducing entity. Why the virus must be inactivated before it becomes an inducer may be that the virus normally synthesizes a protein which acts to block production of interferon by the cell (Sheaff *et al.*, 1972). Inactivation by mild procedures is thought to block the synthesis of this and other viral proteins in preference to viral RNA synthesis.

Reovirus is a virus which contains double-stranded RNA and hence the means by which it induces interferon synthesis might appear to be quite straightforward. A recent study of induction by temperature-sensitive mutants and irradiated reovirus suggests otherwise (Lai and Joklik, 1973). First, it was found that amongst six classes of temperature-sensitive mutants interferon synthesis at the higher temperature failed to correlate with any viral function (including RNA synthesis) except a very late one which resulted in the formation of intact virus particles. Second, a particular mutant which fails to make viral RNA and fails to induce interferon at the higher temperature becomes a potent inducer on irradiation yet RNA synthesis still remains undetectable. It is difficult to interpret these data in a simple manner at the present time.

Another potential difficulty that must be faced by the hypothesis that double-stranded RNA is the universal inducer is that DNA viruses are also interferon inducers. Double-stranded RNA is not thought to be an obligatory intermediate in the replication of these viruses while hybrid double helices consisting of one strand of polydeoxyribonucleotide and one of polyribonucleotide and which are, at least potentially, intermediates, are not effective inducers (section 2.1). However, small amounts of double-stranded viral RNA have been detected in chick cells infected with vaccinia virus, a double-stranded DNA virus, and this RNA might be the component that induces interferon (Colby and Duesberg, 1969). The origin of this double-stranded RNA is obscure; it has been proposed that it results from the transcription of DNA segments located on opposite strands but having a limited extent of overlap (Colby *et al.*, 1971).

Against the argument that double-stranded viral RNA is the effective inducer in the case of vaccinia virus is the finding that vaccinia is in fact a very poor inducer of interferon in chick cells whereas adenovirus, which is a fairly good inducer, fails to yield any double-stranded RNA (Bakay and Burke, 1972). Moreover, irradiation of vaccinia virus, sufficient to inactivate the RNA polymerase in the virus particle which is in part responsible for the synthesis of the double-stranded RNA, results in an increased ability of the virus to induce interferon production. The finding that two temperature-sensitive mutants of adenovirus are defective for interferon induction in chick cells at the nonpermissive temperature may lead to a better understanding of the mechanism of induction by DNA viruses (Ustacelebi and Williams, 1972).

It is apparent that by no means all the data on viral induction of interferon can easily be explained by the hypothesis that double-stranded RNA is the active inducing factor. Three possibilities then suggest themselves. First, it may be that double-stranded RNA really is the active factor in all cases. The lack of correlation between interferon induction and total detectable RNA synthesis or the amount of extractable double-stranded RNA may not be significant since one would suppose that what is important is the amount of double-stranded RNA that is actually present in the cell. Most procedures for detecting intracellular double-stranded RNA involve protein denaturants of one type or another and these are known to convert the nondouble-stranded replicative intermediate to the double-stranded form. Since, as noted earlier, doses of double-stranded polynucleotide corresponding to as little as a few molecules per cell are able to establish antiviral resistance it is certainly conceivable that most viruses could induce sufficient amounts of such RNA to induce interferon synthesis. This RNA would, in general, be regarded as a by-product of the main pathways of macromolecular synthesis and might represent only a very small proportion of the total viral RNA. A further consideration is that the total amount of double-stranded RNA in the cell may be less important than the amount in the vicinity of the specific receptor if this be localized. Animals cells are compartmentalized and different viruses are known to replicate in different compartments.

The second possibility is that there are intracellular receptors for a number of types of viral macromolecules and that interaction between any receptor and the appropriate substrate is sufficient to trigger the synthesis of interferon. Double-stranded RNA might then be a common but not the only viral entity instrumental in induction. A third possibility is that interferon is produced as a nonspecific response to intracellular toxic material. In this case double-stranded RNA would have to exert a very potent toxic effect and indeed there is evidence to support this view (Stinebring and Absher, 1970). At present there is insufficient evidence available to distinguish between the three possible mechanisms for the induction of interferon by viruses.

So far we have considered the mechanisms by which the relatively high potency inducers (double-stranded polynucleotides and viruses) induce interferon. We have also to consider the lower potency inducers which are active primarily in animals but also to some extent in cultures of lymphoid cells. It is known that the *in vitro* exposure of leukocytes to a wide variety of substances including many of the inducers previously described (section 2.2) results in release of a variety of "factors" exerting various biological activities including interferon (Ng and Vilček, 1972). Interferon is released from lymphocytes cultured *in vitro* when these are treated with a nonspecific mitogen such as phytohaemagglutinin (Wheelock, 1965) and from lymphocytes derived from appropriately immune donors in response to treatment with specific bacterial and viral antigens (Green *et al.*, 1969; Epstein *et al.*, 1972). The presence of macrophages augments interferon production by lymphocytes in response to these stimuli (Epstein *et al.*, 1971a and 1971b). It is quite possible that these phenomena may account for the ability of those inducers which clearly do not contain double-stranded RNA to act in the intact animal. Little is known concerning the mechanism by which lymphocytes respond to the variety of interferon inducers of both biological and nonbiological origin.

The final class of interferon inducers to be considered in this section is that of the low molecular weight substances represented by tilorone hydrochloride. There is evidence that this substance may interact with DNA by intercalating its planar ring system between adjacent base-pairs (Chandra *et al.*, 1972). It is not known whether such an interaction is at all related to the interferon inducing ability.

2.4 REGULATION OF INTERFERON SYNTHESIS

The existence of cellular factors which affect the extent of interferon synthesis (section 2.2) implies a degree of control of such synthesis. In particular the existence of the refractory state following induction indicates that interferon synthesis is regulated.

A variety of experiments employing metabolic inhibitors have shed a little light on the mode of control. As noted earlier, if inhibitors of RNA synthesis, such as actinomycin D, or of protein synthesis, such as cycloheximide, are applied to cells at the same time as the inducer then interferon synthesis is blocked. If, however, moderate amounts of such inhibitors are added sometime after the inducer the yield of interferon may be markedly enhanced. Moreover yields are greater if the inhibitor is present only for a limited period and is then removed (Tan *et al.*, 1970; Ng and Vilček, 1972; Vilček and Havell, 1973). The optimum time for addition of the inhibitor appears to depend upon the inducer used. For double-stranded polynucleotides which act rapidly, inhibitors may be added as early as one hour after the inducer but for viruses, which act more slowly, the inhibitor is best added later. Further, there is an optimum dose for each inhibitor such that protein synthesis is not inhibited by more than about 95 per cent. This is of course to be expected since treatment with high doses of inhibitors of protein synthesis would be bound to block further interferon production. Moderate doses of cycloheximide delay the rate of interferon synthesis as well as stimulate the overall level (Vilček and Ng, 1971).

This phenomena of "paradoxical enhancement" or "superinduction" of interferon production by the addition of actinomycin D or cycloheximide late in the induction period has many analogies in other biological systems (Tomkins et al., 1972) and is often interpreted in terms of translational control by a specific repressor (Tomkins et al., 1969). Thus, following induction, the messenger RNA for interferon is made and this is translated to yield interferon. Then it is supposed that the repressor protein is made and this blocks translation of the interferon messenger. Inhibitors of protein or RNA synthesis added shortly after induction are presumed to block the synthesis of the repressor either directly or by inhibiting the synthesis of its messenger RNA. The synthesis of the repressor must be more sensitive to the effects of the inhibitors than is the synthesis of interferon. It is possible, though not demonstrated, that this putative repressor protein is responsible for the establishment of the refractory state following induction.

It should be stressed that the above model for interferon "superinduction" is speculative and other interpretations of the data are possible. For example, if the messenger RNA for interferon was more stable than most other cellular messengers then, following actinomycin treatment, the proportion of interferon messenger present in the cell would increase; if messenger RNA was normally present in excess then the rate of interferon synthesis would increase. This type of explanation has been proposed for other systems (Palmiter and Schimke, 1973).

A line of mouse fibroblasts transformed by a murine sarcoma virus has been described which may lack the interferon regulatory system (Chany and Vignal, 1970). These cells produced interferon following five sequential challenges with Newcastle Disease virus during a 48-hour period. It is possible therefore that the normal control mechanism is deficient. However, because these cells are also quite insensitive to interferon treatment an alternative hypothesis in which interferon itself feeds back to inhibit its own synthesis has been proposed (Colby and Morgan, 1971).

3   Purification and properties of interferon

3.1   PURIFICATION OF INTERFERON

As starting material for the purification of interferon, substantial amounts of infected cell material are required. Most commonly, cell cultures infected with a good viral inducer are used. For example, L cells infected with irradiated Newcastle Disease virus have been used as starting material for the purification of mouse interferon (Paucker *et al.*, 1970), while human leukocytes, derived as a by-product of a Blood Transfusion Service, may be infected *in vitro* to yield quantities of human interferon (Strander and Cantell, 1966; Strander *et al.*, 1973). Allantoic fluids derived from chick embryos infected with influenza virus (a by-product of vaccine manufacture) have been used as the starting material for extensive purification of chick interferon (Fantes, 1967). In order to simplify the purification process it has been found possible in certain cases to omit the usual requirement of serum from the medium (Paucker *et al.*, 1970; Tovey *et al.*, 1973). Techniques that offer the possibility of enhancing interferon yields include the use of antimetabolites following induction (section 2.4), the use of "priming" by pretreatment with small quantities of interferon (section 4.3) and the use of cell lines which produce exceptionally large amounts of interferon (section 2.2).

A wide variety of methods have been employed for the purification of interferon. Because a completely pure preparation of any one type has not knowingly been obtained there is no one standard set of procedures that can be recommended. A few of the more commonly used techniques of protein chemistry that have been applied to the purification of interferon will now be mentioned. Fuller discussions are available (Ng and Vilček, 1972; Fantes, 1973).

Concentration of the initial fluids can be achieved by reversible absorption to a variety of materials, by precipitation with ammonium sulphate, or by using the recent technique of ultrafiltration through membranes of specific pore size. Purification procedures include the use of low pH to denature many contaminant proteins but not interferon, and, most usefully, ion-exchange chromatography on DEAE- or CM-cellulose (or the equivalent Sephadex derivatives). Electrophoresis and isoelectric focusing in a variety of support media, including polyacrylamide gels, have been used, usually at the later stages of a purification to avoid problems of overloading. These techniques are limited, however, by the charge heterogeneity of interferon (section 3.2). Gel filtration on Sephadex has been used in the purification of interferon but the size heterogeneity of interferon (see below) limits the usefulness of this method preparatively. Analytically, however, it is of great importance (section 3.2).

A newer and very convenient method of protein purification that is currently being applied to the purification of interferon is affinity chromatography (Sipe *et al.*, 1973; Ogburn *et al.*, 1973). Here, antiserum is raised against the interferon preparation of greatest purity conveniently available and this is covalently attached to a solid support material. Passage of a crude interferon preparation over such material results in the specific absorption of the interferon which can subsequently be eluted. Best results are obtained if the anti-interferon serum is first absorbed against preparations of the contaminant viral and cellular proteins before attachment to the solid phase.

The chick interferon preparation of highest purity is probably that of Fantes (1967) with specific activity of 1.6×10^6 units per mg protein. Acrylamide gel electrophoresis indicated that most of the protein in the preparation was not related to the antiviral activity (Fantes and Furminger, 1967). Mouse interferon preparations with specific activity of 3×10^7 international reference units per mg protein have been prepared by a procedure involving preparative electrophoresis as the final step (Paucker et al., 1970; Stanček and Paucker, 1971). Recently the use of affinity chromatography has enabled a specific activity of 2.7×10^8 units per mg to be reached (Ogburn et al., 1973). Rabbit interferon has been purified to a specific activity of 4.8×10^7 units per mg protein (Yamazaki and Wagner, 1970). The purification of human interferon has progressed less far. There appears to be no detailed account of an extensive purification in the recent literature, though material of specific activity $2–6 \times 10^6$ units per mg protein has been reported (Fantes, 1970; Mogensen and Cantell, 1974). It should be said that the relative degree of purity of interferons from different species cannot be judged on the basis of specific activity data since this depends on the sensitivity of the assay system employed or on the arbitrary units of international reference preparations.

It would be useful to have available radioactively labelled interferon particularly for studies on its mode of action. Attempts have been made to prepare and purify such material (Paucker et al., 1970; Yamazaki and Wagner, 1970) but since the purity of the preparations is unknown the proportion of the radioactive label that represents interferon is equally uncertain.

Analysis of crude or partially purified interferon preparation will usually indicate the presence of biologically active components having a range of molecular weights and isoelectric points (see section 3.2). Thus some workers prefer to speak of the interferons in the plural. Even when a preparation has been fractionated to remove size and charge heterogeneity so that there is no detectable form of inhomogeneity one cannot make any strong statement about purity. A theoretical approach may, however, be adopted. On the assumption that one interferon molecule is sufficient to protect a single cell against infection it has been calculated that the minimum number of molecules required to give 50 per cent protection in a typical assay (i.e. one unit of activity) would be about 1.4×10^6 (Ng and Vilček, 1972). If the molecular weight of interferon is taken to be 30 000 then the specific activity of the pure material would be about 2.5×10^9 units per mg protein. If, as is probable, more than one molecule of interferon is required to effect detectable protection of a cell (say ten) then the specific activity of the pure material would be reduced correspondingly (say to 2.5×10^8 units per mg). This last figure is close to the best preparations currently available. Thus one may hope for good progress in the near future on the complete purification and chemical characterization of the interferon molecule.

3.2 PHYSICOCHEMICAL PROPERTIES OF INTERFERON

Since interferon of known purity has not been available experiments on the physicochemical properties of the substance have been restricted to those cases where the biological activity may be followed. Despite this limitation a good deal of information has been obtained (Ng and Vilček, 1972; Fantes, 1973). The stability of interferon preparations is variable but may be high. Preparations of chick interferon may be stable to heating at 70°C for 1 hour though most other interferons are less resistant. A very characteristic property of interferon is stability over a wide pH range. A large measure of stability at pH 2 is one of the standard properties of all species while stability from pH1 to 10 is usual. Moreover, it appears that both mouse and human interferon preparations are substantially more resistant to heat inactivation (37°C or 56°C) at pH 3·5 than at pH 7·0 (Marshall *et al.*, 1972). Recently, it was found that interferon can be renatured after denaturation in a boiling mixture of sodium dodecyl sulphate, thioethanol and urea (Stewart, 1974). Interferon preparations are usually reasonably resistant to freezing and thawing and to freeze-drying.

Losses of the biological activity of a preparation may be experienced and this is especially true of highly purified preparations. Such losses may be attributed, at least in part, to adsorption to surfaces. Plastic containers may be more suitable than glass when this problem is experienced. To obviate the loss of activity it is common to add a carrier protein, usually bovine serum albumin, before the final stages of a purification procedure. However this will obviously not be possible when chemical characterization becomes feasible.

The activity of interferon is irreversibly destroyed by treatment with proteolytic enzymes such as trypsin but is not affected by other enzymes that have been tested such as ribo-and deoxyribonucleases, and lipases. This is the main reason for believing interferon to be a protein. Consistent with this is the finding that biological activity is lost following reduction by mercaptoethanol but can be recovered completely if the reduced interferon molecule is unfolded in the presence of urea or guanidine hydrochloride and then allowed to oxidize in air (Mogensen and Cantell, 1974). This suggests that at least one disulphide bond is important for biological activity.

Interferon, like most proteins secreted by cells, is a glycoprotein. The carbohydrate moiety terminates in one or more sialic acid residues attached to a galactose residue (Dorner *et al.*, 1973). The sialic acid residues can be removed by treatment with neuraminidase without loss of biological activity.

The most extensively investigated property of interferon is its molecular weight. The usual technique for measuring this is by gel filtration on a Sephadex column which has been calibrated with known proteins. Molecular weight values are commonly in the range 20 000 to 30 000 but values of up to 160 000 have been reported (for a tabulation of data see Ng and Vilček, 1972). A given preparation often contains more than one molecular weight species. When interferon is induced in animals the molecular weight may also depend upon the nature of the inducer. It is not known if a given cell can produce more than one molecular weight species or whether different cell types are responsible.

The existence of interferon species of different size may be explained in three ways. First, they may consist of quite distinct molecular entities, the only common property being their biological activity. Second, there may exist a relatively small active molecule which may be bound to various types of carrier protein. Third, the larger species may be oligomers of a smaller subunit. Evidence in support of this last hypothesis has been reported by Carter (1970) who was able to separate by isoelectric focusing mouse interferon species of molecular weights of 19 000 and 38 000 and human interferon species of 12 000 and 24 000. Conversion of the larger to the smaller forms was possible by reducing the ionic strength but the reverse conversion has not been achieved. Larger species might be dimers of the smaller but Stewart (1974) concluded from analysis by electrophoresis under denaturing conditions that two mouse interferons were distinct entities.

Although some preparations of interferon display relatively simple patterns following isoelectric focusing (Carter, 1970), in other cases multiple components have been reported (Fantes, 1969; Schonne *et al.*, 1970). This indicates the presence of heterogeneity with respect to charge. Treatment with neuraminidase was found to generate one major component (Schonne *et al.*, 1970; Dorner *et al.*, 1973) and this suggested that the charge heterogeneity is due to a variable degree of glycosylation. Consistent with this was the finding that when sialic acid residues were attached enzymically to the neuraminidase-treated molecule the original change heterogeneity was recovered (Dorner *et al.*, 1973).

As would be expected interferon is antigenic (Levy-Koenig *et al.*, 1970a). The use of interferon antiserum as a means of purifying interferon was noted in the previous section.

4 Action of interferon

4.1 GENERAL ASPECTS OF THE ANTIVIRAL ACTION OF INTERFERON

In general cells must be incubated with interferon for some time prior to challenge with the virus if an inhibition of virus growth is to be seen. Detectable resistance to infection develops more rapidly when larger doses of interferon are used but the time at which the maximum extent of resistance is reached seems to be independent of the dose and is about 8 h in mouse cells (Baron *et al.*, 1967). Development of resistance to viral infection occurs when cells and interferon are incubated at 37°C but to a far smaller extent when incubated at 4°C.

The degree of resistance to virus growth is directly related to the doses of interferon employed. The dose–response curve is sigmoidal when, as is customary, the concentration of interferon is expressed logarithmically. There is an obvious analogy with the simplest model for drug–receptor interaction, which assumes that a tissue possesses a population of identical and noninteracting receptors for a particular drug, and which yields a sigmoidal dose–response curve on the further assumption that the effect produced is proportional to the fraction of receptors occupied (Rang, 1971). Experimental values for the slope of the dose–response curve at the central line portion have been interpreted as indicating that one molecule of interferon is sufficient to protect a cell from infection (Gifford and Koch, 1969).

Some curious results have been obtained with monkey–mouse hybrid cells which are sensitive to both primate and mouse interferons (Chany *et al.*, 1973). When mouse interferon was assayed in the hybrid cells or in parental mouse cells the dose–response curves were sigmoidal and parallel, but when primate interferon was assayed the slope of the curve found for the hybrid cells was substantially less than that for parental monkey cells. The experiments were taken to indicate the existence of an "activator", which would promote the uptake of interferon, in addition to the receptor for the interferon molecule. This view is quite speculative, however.

The effect of interferon is to slow the rate of virus replication thereby reducing the yield at any particular time compared with that of untreated cells. The reduction in yield due to a given dose of interferon may therefore depend on the time of harvesting and will usually be maximal when the yield from the untreated control cells has just reached its peak. A cell culture will retain its resistance to virus infection while interferon remains present in the medium but when it is removed resistance is lost over a period of time. In the case of mouse cells, it has been reported that full sensitivity was not regained until about 48 h after the removal of interferon (Baron *et al.*, 1967).

The titre of an interferon preparation appears to be independent of the dose of challenge virus employed (Hallum and Youngner, 1966). It may, however, be dependent on the nature of the virus used in the assay. Each species of interferon appears to have its own characteristic spectrum of activity against different types of viruses. Thus in one study vaccinia virus was the most sensitive of five viruses tested using hamster and mouse interferons but was the least sensitive with human and rabbit interferons, while, conversely, Semliki forest virus (an arbovirus) was the least sensitive to hamster and mouse interferons but was relatively sensitive to rabbit interferon (Stewart et al., 1969). In another study, SV40 and polyoma virus, two very similar, small DNA viruses, were found to differ in sensitivity to mouse interferon by a factor of at least 150 (Oxman and Takemoto, 1970).

The relative sensitivity of two viruses to a given interferon may be dependent on the type of assay employed. Thus when the sensitivities of Newcastle Disease virus (NDV) and Vesicular Stomatitis virus (VSV) to chick interferon in chick cells were compared by the plaque reduction assay, which involves multiple cycles of cirus replication, they were found to differ by a factor of 45, whereas in a single-cycle yield inhibition assay no difference in sensitivity was found (Hallum et al., 1970). This result was explained by the finding that resistance to NDV, the less sensitive virus, decayed more rapidly than resistance to VSV. Thus when an assay which involves multiple cycles of virus replication is used the rate of decay of the antiviral effect may be as important as the inherent sensitivity of the virus to interferon in determining the apparent sensitivity. This may, in part, account for some of the differences in sensitivity of different viruses to interferon referred to in the previous paragraph. To make a rather broad generalization, the arboviruses and VSV are usually considered most sensitive to interferon while the herpes and adenovirus groups are considered the least sensitive.

Interferon is usually described as being species specific. That is, mouse interferon, for example, is active only in mouse cells and not in cells of other species, but there are some well-established exceptions to this rule. For example human interferon is active in monkey cells (Bucknall, 1967) and may be even more active in rabbit cells than in human cells (Desmyter et al., 1968). It is interesting that the effect of human interferon in rabbit cells is neutralized by an antiserum to rabbit interferon, suggesting the presence of common antigenic components in interferons of the two species (Levy-Koenig et al., 1970b). Another exception to the general rule is that monkey interferon protects rat cells though human, mouse and rabbit interferons do not (Uhlendorf et al., 1973). In view of these exceptions the species specificity of interferon is best described as being characteristic rather than absolute. Interferon does not appear to be tissue specific (Riley and Gifford, 1967).

While interferon inhibits virus growth it does not necessarily prevent cell destruction. Thus mouse interferon can inhibit substantially the multiplication of both vaccinia virus and Mengo virus in mouse L cells yet in both cases the cells are completely destroyed (Joklik and Merigan, 1966; Gauntt and Lockart, 1968). With considerably higher doses of interferon, however, protection against cell destruction has been reported (Haase *et al.*, 1969). The mechanism of this cytopathic effect is not well understood. Although interferon treatment may not save an individual infected cell from destruction it does reduce the yield of virus from such a cell and thereby reduces the spread of infection through the population.

Little interferon need absorb to cells to induce antiviral resistance. Indeed, in some experiments no detectable loss of activity from the culture fluids has been observed (Buckler *et al.*, 1966). Where loss of activity has been found this may often have been due to nonspecific absorption or to enzymic digestion. In some cases, however, it has been possible to recover interferon from cells to which it has been bound (Sheaff and Stewart, 1969; Stewart *et al.*, 1972a). The specificity of the binding is suggested by the fact that elution only occurred from cells of the same species as the interferon and not from heterologous cells.

Resistance to viral infection is not manifested when cells are incubated with interferon in the cold (1°C). When, after such an incubation, the cells are washed and then incubated at 37°C for a period the antiviral effect is seen (Friedman, 1967). If, before transfer to 37°C, the cells are exposed to trypsin the development of resistance is inhibited. These results suggest that interferon is bound to a surface receptor in the cold but that a period at 37°C is required for the development of resistance. While attachment of interferon to cells appears to be necessary, nothing is known about the nature of the interaction. It is not clear if interferon has to penetrate into the cell for the antiviral effect to develop or whether it need only bind to an appropriate surface receptor. Interferon covalently bound to a solid support is active, suggesting that the receptor is at the cell surface (Ankel *et al.*, 1973; Knight, 1974; Chany *et al.*, 1974). It is possible, however, that this activity is due to a small amount of interferon that is released from the support when in contact with the cells.

A variety of factors affect the action of interferon (Vilček, 1969; Sonnabend and Friedman, 1973). These include the age of the cells, the pH, and a number of little characterized factors derived from cell culture media, cell extracts or from serum which antagonize or enhance the effect of interferon. Metabolic inhibitors also interfere with the action of interferon and these will be discussed in the following section.

4.2 MECHANISM OF ACTION OF INTERFERON

This section falls into three parts. First, we consider the nature of the intracellular events that lead to the establishment of the antiviral state. Second, evidence relating to the stage(s) in the viral replication cycle that is blocked by the interferon-mediated inhibition is reviewed. Third, what is known of the molecular basis for the inhibition is described.

Most of our knowledge concerning the events leading to the establishment of the state of resistance to virus infection comes from studies with metabolic inhibitors. There is good evidence that cellular RNA synthesis is required for this process. If cellular RNA synthesis is blocked by actinomycin D during the interferon treatment no resistance to infection develops (Taylor, 1964). For this type of experiment an RNA virus which is insensitive to actinomycin D is employed to assay the antiviral state of the cells. Thus the drug can be present throughout the experiment and there is no need to reverse its effect in order to permit virus growth. It is generally assumed that the effect of actinomycin D in the above experiment is to block the synthesis of messenger RNA coding for a protein having intracellular antiviral activity (the "antiviral protein"). There is, however, as yet no direct evidence that the RNA whose synthesis is required is mRNA.

It has been argued that the required RNA is unlikely to be ribosomal since the lowest dose of actinomycin which almost completely abolished the effect of interferon still permitted some ribosomal RNA synthesis to occur (Friedman, 1970). Studies using enucleated cells are consistent with the above ideas. Removal of nuclei prior to interferon treatment does not render the cells resistant to infection while enucleation after treatment does not reduce the antiviral effect (Radke et al., 1974).

Similar experiments to those described above have been attempted using inhibitors of protein synthesis in order to determine whether this is required for the establishment of the interferon-induced antiviral state. The results are less convincing since it is necessary to reverse the effect of the drug in order to permit virus growth during the assay of the resistant state. Furthermore, some inhibitors of protein synthesis may affect RNA synthesis, probably through a secondary mechanism, and this will make the result difficult to interpret. Nevertheless, studies with a number of inhibitors do suggest that development of resistance in response to interferon may have a requirement for cellular protein synthesis (Sonnabend et al., 1970). On the other hand, at least one effective inhibitor of protein synthesis, cycloheximide, appears not to block the action of interferon (Dianzani et al., 1969). This result was rationalized by postulating that mRNA for the antiviral protein is made in the presence of the inhibitor of protein synthesis and is then translated when this inhibitor is washed out prior to infection. If this is the case it is not clear why the same argument should not apply to the other inhibitors of protein synthesis that have been employed and where an inhibition of the effect of interferon has been seen (Sonnabend *et al.*, 1970).

Thus although it is widely believed that cellular protein synthesis is necessary for the antiviral effect of interferon to be manifest the available evidence is by no means as compelling as one would like. Moreover, although the existence of a specific antiviral protein and its mRNA are generally assumed the possibility that it is merely the continuation of normal cellular RNA and protein synthesis that is required has not been excluded. For example, if interferon were itself directly antiviral within the cell, its uptake into the cell might require cellular RNA and protein synthesis. While making these reservations, however, we shall assume the existence of an antiviral protein whose synthesis is induced by interferon during the remainder of this discussion. The finding that a specific human gene is required if human–mouse hybrid cell lines are to show sensitivity to human interferon is consistent with the existence of a cellular protein whose synthesis is induced by interferon. This gene maps on chromosome G-21 (Tan *et al.*, 1973).

Once the antiviral state is established it cannot be reversed by metabolic inhibitors. Indeed treatment with actinomycin D after substantial resistance to infection has been established may result in an enhancement of the antiviral effect (Chany *et al.*, 1971). This result has been taken to indicate the existence of a regulatory protein that controls the antiviral state in a manner perhaps analogous to the regulatory protein that is thought to control interferon synthesis (see section 2.4).

There is one item of evidence which suggests that, in addition to interferon treatment, virus infection may also be required to establish the antiviral effect. As will be described later in this section, it has been possible to prepare a cell-free protein synthesizing system which appears to display an interferon-mediated inhibition of the translation of exogenous encephalomyocarditis (EMC) virus RNA *in vitro* (Friedman *et al.*, 1972). To do this it was found necessary not only to treat the cells from which the *in vitro* extract was made with interferon but also to infect them with virus (e.g. vaccinia virus). This suggests that treatment of cells with interferon alone may lead to the establishment of a latent antiviral state which is "triggered" to the fully active state by infection. This possibility was only raised when a *in vitro* assay (i.e. using cell extracts) for the effect of interferon became possible, since detection of the antiviral state *in vivo* of course requires virus infection of the cells.

We now consider the stage(s) in the replication cycle of the virus that is inhibited by interferon. Interferon inhibits viral replication in cells inoculated with infectious RNA isolated from a number of viruses (Vikček, 1969). This indicates that absorption or penetration of the virus particle into the cell is not the stage at which the interferon mechanism acts. There is extensive evidence (see below) that the synthesis of new viral nucleic acid is prevented by interferon treatment and thus the locus of action is prior to maturation of the progeny virus particle. Our attention focuses, therefore, on viral macromolecular synthesis.

Picornaviruses and arboviruses are single-stranded RNA viruses that contain within the virus particle no enzymic activity. The RNA of the virus particle that infects the cell acts initially as messenger RNA which codes for the synthesis of viral RNA polymerase activity. This enzyme utilizes the same input strand of RNA as a template for the synthesis of new RNA strands which may act as new messenger, as new template or as viral RNA within the progeny virus particles. An intermediate in the synthesis of new single-stranded RNA is a replicative form consisting of a strand of viral RNA, its complementary copy and the RNA polymerase enzyme. When this replicative form is isolated under conditions of protein denaturation double-stranded RNA is obtained.

The effect of interferon treatment is to inhibit the formation of viral RNA whether measured by the incorporation of radioactive precursors or as infectious RNA after extraction from the cells. The synthesis of all forms of intracellular viral RNA is inhibited, including the double-stranded replicative form, in Semliki Forest virus-infected chick cells (Mecs et al., 1967). The incorporation of the RNA of the infecting virus particle into this double-stranded form has also been shown to be inhibited by interferon treatment (Friedman et al., 1967). Inhibition of viral RNA synthesis could be due to the inhibition of the action of the RNA polymerase or to inhibition of the synthesis of this enzyme. Interferon treatment resulted in reduced levels of viral RNA polymerase activity in infected cells, as expected, and the failure to detect an inhibitor of polymerase activity in extracts of interferon treated cells led to the suggestion that it was the synthesis of the viral enzyme (and probably of all viral proteins) that was blocked (Sonnabend et al., 1967). Of course the failure to detect an inhibitor of polymerase activity in an in vitro assay is not conclusive since it might have been unstable or inaccessible. In support of the proposal that interferon inhibits viral protein synthesis in general is the finding that interferon treatment markedly reduces the synthesis of all five polypeptides coded by what is thought to be the RNA of the input Semliki Forest virus particle (Friedman, 1968).

A number of animal viruses containing a single-stranded RNA genome also contain RNA polymerase enzymic activity within the virus particle.

In these cases it appears that the initial event of the replication cycle in the infected cell is the transcription of the viral RNA by the virion polymerase. The transcript is complementary to the virus RNA strand and is the message which codes for the viral proteins. Vesicular stomatitis virus (VSV) is a virus of this type and the effect of interferon pretreatment of the functioning of the viral polymerase in infected cells has been described (Marcus et al., 1971; Manders et al., 1972). It was claimed that interferon inhibits the activity of this polymerase and thus the transcription of viral RNA is inhibited in this system. A similar situation has been suggested for influenza-virus infected cells (Bean and Simpson, 1973). However, a recent reinvestigation of these two virus-cell systems has led to the conclusion that interferon does not, in fact, inhibit transcription by the varion polymerase but, rather, may block viral protein synthesis (Repik et al., 1974).

We now turn to the DNA viruses, and here vaccinia virus has been most extensively studied with respect to the site of action of interferon. Vaccinia virus, a member of the pox virus group, is a large virus with a double-stranded DNA genome, and RNA polymerase activity within the particle, and a somewhat complicated structure. On entry into the cell the outer envelope is lost (this is known as "first-stage uncoating") and the core of the virus is liberated into the cytoplasm of the cell. This core contains the DNA genome and the polymerase which is then activated and this results in a burst of viral mRNA synthesis which codes for early viral proteins (Metz and Esteban, 1972). Viral DNA is subsequently liberated from the core structure ("second-stage uncoating") and then viral DNA replication occurs.

The effect of interferon on vaccinia replication is to inhibit viral DNA synthesis (Joklik and Merigan, 1966) and to block second-stage uncoating so that viral cores accumulate in the cytoplasm of the infected cell (Magee et al., 1968). Inhibitors of protein synthesis such as cycloheximide also inhibit viral DNA synthesis and second-stage uncoating. Interferon treatment results in a significant enhancement of early viral RNA synthesis in the infected cell which is effected by the viron polymerase (Joklik and Merigan, 1966; Jungwirth et al., 1972; Metz and Esteban, 1972). Inhibitors of protein synthesis also enhance viral RNA synthesis and it is presumed that one of the proteins normally synthesized under the direction of this mRNA acts to switch off viral RNA synthesis. Hence if protein synthesis is blocked this switch-off does not occur. The similarity between the effects of inhibitors of protein synthesis and of interferon suggested that interferon may be blocking viral protein synthesis. This has been directly demonstrated at times as early as 30 minutes after infection (Metz and Esteban, 1972).

Investigations of the fate of the vaccinia viral mRNA, which is transcribed but does not appear to be translated, show that its ability to associate with the ribosomes to form functional polyribosomes is diminished (Joklik and Merigan, 1966). It appears that both the initiation of viral polypeptide chain synthesis and chain elongation are inhibited and that the interaction of a viral mRNA-protein complex with the small ribosomal subunit is the stage at which initiation is blocked (Metz et al., 1975).

Thus in the case of vaccinia virus infection it seems reasonably clear that interferon inhibits viral translation but not viral transcription, though there is one report which suggests that transcription may be inhibited in this system (Bialy and Colby, 1972; cf. Metz and Esteban, 1972, and Esteban and Metz, 1973).

SV40 is a small DNA-containing virus of considerable current interest since it is able to cause the morphological transformation of certain types of cells and may therefore be described as an oncogenic agent. In permissive cells (e.g. monkey cells) the virus replicates normally while in nonpermissive cells (e.g. mouse cells) no infectious virus is produced but a proportion of the cells may be transformed. Interferon pretreatment of the 3T3 line of mouse cells inhibits transformation of these cells by SV40 (Todaro and Baron, 1965). Moreover, interferon pretreatment blocks the synthesis of the SV40 early protein known as the T antigen and which is made both in permissive cells and in nonpermissive cells prior to their becoming transformed (Oxman and Black, 1966). T antigen is also synthesized in lines of cells which are transformed by SV40 but are free of detectable virus and where it is believed that the SV40 genome is integrated into that of the host cells. It is particularly interesting that in such transformed cells T antigen production is entirely insensitive to interferon treatment (Oxman et al., 1967a) and this suggests that the portion of the viral genome that is recognized by the interferon mechanism is inoperative in this situation. It cannot be missing since normal, infectious SV40 virus can be recovered from such transformed lines by an appropriate manipulation.

A variety of adenovirus-SV40 hybrid viruses have been prepared in the laboratory in which a portion of the SV40 is inserted into the larger adenovirus DNA genome. In some of these both the SV40 T antigen and the adenovirus T antigen, which is similar to but immunologically distinguishable from the SV40 antigen, are expressed. Now adenovirus is relatively resistant to interferon treatment (being about 100-fold less sensitive than SV40) and it was found that in the hybrid viruses SV40 T antigen synthesis showed a resistance to interferon quantitatively indistinguishable from that of adenovirus T antigens (Oxman et al., 1967b). Thus, just as in the case of the SV40 transformed cells, in the hybrid viruses the portion of the SV40 genome that is recognized by the interferon mechanism is inoperative or absent. These results suggested that there might exist in cells infected by the adenovirus-SV40 hybrid virus a hybrid mRNA containing both adenovirus and SV40 sequences covalently linked and indeed the existence of such an RNA species has recently been detected (Oxman *et al.*, 1974).

The effect of interferon treatment on the synthesis of early SV40 RNA, which is presumed to code for the T antigen and other early viral proteins, has been investigated (Oxman and Levin, 1971). It was found that the synthesis of this RNA was inhibited which suggested that interferon acted to block the transcription of viral RNA in this system.

Before considering the implications of these various findings on the site of action of the interferon mechanism we must first discuss the question of whether viral functions are specifically discriminated against in interferon-treated, infected cells. It is clear that there is no inhibition of gross RNA or protein synthesis in uninfected cells which have been treated with doses of interferon sufficient to inhibit the growth of a reasonably sensitive virus by 99 per cent (more subtle, qualitative changes in RNA and protein synthesis cannot be ruled out, however, and there is some evidence that inhibition can occur at higher doses; see section 4.3). As discussed earlier, however, there is some evidence that the antiviral effect of interferon is not fully manifested in uninfected cells, infection being required to "trigger" the effect. Hence RNA and protein synthesis in interferon-treated, uninfected cells may not be a proper measure of cellular RNA and protein synthesis in interferon-treated, infected cells. Estimation of the effect of interferon on cellular macromolecular synthesis in infected cells is not straightforward since many viruses are able to shut off cellular synthetic functions. This may occur in a variety of ways. In the case of vaccinia virus, for example, a component of the infecting particle inhibits cellular protein synthesis and this occurs in both interferon-treated as well as in untreated cells (Metz and Esteban, 1972). Thus it is not possible to determine whether interferon treatment has any effect on cellular protein synthesis in vaccinia infected cells. Obviously what is required is a virus which does not shut off cellular macromolecular synthesis. SV40 is such a virus and in interferon-treated SV40 infected cells one finds that viral RNA and T antigen synthesis are inhibited while the synthesis of total cellular RNA, of cellular RNA that hybridizes to cellular DNA and of total cellular proteins are not affected (Oxman and Levin, 1971; Metz and Oxman, unpublished observations). This suggests that the interferon-mediated inhibition of SV40 RNA synthesis is specific and is not due to a general inhibition of all RNA synthesis. The possibility that the synthesis of some cellular mRNA species is inhibited in this situation has not been eliminated. There is no well-documented example of interferon-mediated inhibition of viral translation in the case of a virus that does not shut off cellular protein synthesis and hence we do not know if the inhibition of translation is virus specific, although there are indirect suggestions that this is indeed the case (Gupta *et al.*, 1974). Taking all the available evidence into account it seems probable that the effect of interferon is to inhibit specifically viral and not cellular macromolecular synthesis in infected cells. The alternative possibility that infection of the interferon-treated and latently antiviral cell triggers a generalized shutdown of all macromolecular synthesis is therefore unlikely, although it is a conceptually simpler and biologically not implausible model.

We have reviewed the best studied cases that bear on the question of the point in the viral replication cycle at which the interferon mechanism acts. As we have seen there is evidence that both virus transcription and translation may be inhibited, depending on the virus-cell system examined. Although there is no direct evidence on the point it would not be surprising if transcription and translation were inhibited in the same infected cell. One type of explanation for these findings is that there are distinct intracellular inhibitors of viral transcription and of translation. This would not seem to be biologically unreasonable since if for any reason one of these processes was insensitive to the inhibition the other would still be susceptible. For example, in the case of vaccinia virus early RNA made within the intracellular viral core is not inhibited in interferon-treated cells and this may be because the core is impermeable to macromolecules as small as the drug actinomycin D (Metz and Esteban, 1972).

A second type of explanation, which is somewhat more economical, is to postulate that a single intracellular entity can inhibit both viral transcription and translation. Here one might suppose that the antiviral protein is able to discriminate between cellular and viral nucleic acids (whether DNA or RNA) and to bind to the latter, thereby blocking their function, whether as template or as message. The conceptual difficulty that we have with both types of hypotheses is the problem of discrimination between viral and cellular DNA or RNA. We shall return to this question at the end of this section.

There is some indirect evidence for the existence of more than one intracellular inhibitor. In interferon-treated chick cells resistance to NDV appears to decay more rapidly than does resistance to VSV, suggesting that distinct factors are involved (Hallum *et al.*, 1970). Pseudorabies virus (a herpes virus) and vaccinia virus are as susceptible as VSV to interferon when tested in chick or mouse cells but in rabbit cells they are far less sensitive (Youngner *et al.*, 1972). Moreover, in doubly infected rabbit cells VSV replication is inhibited by interferon while pseudorabies replication is refractory.

While these results are suggestive, a proper understanding of whether there are single or multiple intracellular inhibitors and of their modes of action will only come when we are able to study these events in cell-free systems. If we have *in vitro* systems in which interferon-mediated inhibition of viral transcription and translation can be demonstrated then we can attempt to purify the inhibitory factors and to determine whether the factor from the transcription system inhibits in the translation system and vice versa. Appropriate cell-free translation systems for the study of the interferon effect have been developed and to these we now turn our attention. As yet no interferon-mediated inhibition in an *in vitro* transcription system has been demonstrated.

An *in vitro* translation system from an animal cell may utilize a relatively crude post-mitochondrial supernatant preparation; this may be further fractionated and purified into ribosomes and a variety of initiation factors, elongation factors, transfer RNAs etc. To this is added appropriate co-factors and amino acids, at least one of which is radioactive, and a messenger RNA. This mRNA may be of viral origin, such as encephalomyocarditis virus RNA (EMC RNA), or cellular, such as globin mRNA purified from reticulocytes. After incubation the radioactive polypeptides that are made must be characterized in order to demonstrate that their synthesis was coded by the added mRNA.

The behaviour of such *in vitro* systems depends on the mode of preparation of the extracts and on the conditions of assay and this is especially true when one is trying to demonstrate regulation of translation *in vitro*. Thus before considering the results of *in vitro* studies we will discuss experiments in which the fate of the viral messenger RNA in interferon-treated, infected cells has been examined. These should indicate the behaviour to be expected from the cell-free systems.

Vaccinia virus provides a good model system for such studies since, as noted earlier, viral mRNA is extensively synthesized by the RNA polymerase of the infecting particle even in interferon-treated cells. The association of this RNA with cellular ribosomes to form viral polyribosomes is partially inhibited in interferon-treated cells (Joklik and Merigan, 1966), and this is due to a diminished rate of initiation of viral polypeptide synthesis (Metz *et al.*, 1975). Moreover, the rate of elongation of viral polypeptide chains is also reduced. The inhibition of initiation appears to be due to the decreased ability of the small ribosomal subunit to associate with the viral mRNA. The fact that polypeptide chain elongation is inhibited as well as chain initiation suggests that interferon does not simply modify message-specific initiation factors. Rather, the situation is reminiscent of that found in the case of a number of antibiotic inhibitors of protein synthesis which act by binding to one of the ribosomal subunits and often inhibit chain initiation more than elongation or vice versa. These, of course do not discriminate between viral and cellular protein synthesis.

Another approach to the study of the effect of interferon on the viral mRNA in the intact cell is to follow the fate of the radioactively labelled RNA of a single stranded RNA virus, such as a picorna- or arbovirus, which acts as a messenger immediately after the uncoating of the virus particle in the infected cell. This approach is technically quite difficult. Levy and Carter (1968) claimed that the RNA of Mengo virus formed a complex with the small ribosomal subunit soon after infection and that interferon treatment blocked this process. However, interpretation of this result is difficult because only a very small proportion of the RNA of the infecting virus was found in the complex which itself was poorly characterized.

The earliest *in vitro* studies on the effect of interferon pretreatment on virus translation were those of Marcus and Salb (1966). They claimed that ribosomes from interferon-treated cells could combine with, but not translate, viral RNA, though they could still translate cellular mRNA. Some reduction in the affinity of interferon-treated cell ribosomes for viral RNA was also observed. Carter and Levy (1967) found a more pronounced reduction in binding of viral RNA to ribosomes from interferon-treated cells. These results, however, have not been reproduced in other laboratories and thus their status remains in doubt, especially in view of poor characterization of the viral RNA-ribosome complexes (Kerr *et al.*, 1970; Kerr, 1971; Colby and Morgan, 1971).

Recently a cell-free system has been developed in which the synthesis of EMC virus polypeptides in mouse L cell in response to added EMC RNA is inhibited when the extracts are prepared from cells treated with relatively low doses of interferon and then infected with virus (Friedman *et al.*, 1972). Extracts from cells treated with interferon but not infected, or from untreated, infected cells displayed little if any decrease in activity. Infection with both vaccinia virus and EMC virus "triggers" the apparently latent antiviral state. The interesting feature of this cell-free system is the requirement for virus infection prior to preparation of the cell extracts. This is not unreasonable biologically since of course the antiviral state is not required to be operative until the infecting virus enters the cell. Both the initiation of viral polypeptide synthesis and chain elongation are inhibited in extracts from interferon-treated cells, the former effect predominating (Kerr *et al.*, 1974a). This is in agreement with the studies on vaccinia polypeptide synthesis in intact, interferon-treated cells, as noted earlier.

Cell-free systems which display an interferon-mediated inhibition of translation without prior infection have also been prepared (Kerr, 1971; Falcoff *et al.*, 1972; Falcoff *et al.*, 1973; Gupta *et al.*, 1973; Samuel and Joklik, 1974). It is not entirely clear at present how these differ from the infected-cell system described above. It is possible that the way in which the cells are manipulated or the extracts prepared produces an effect analogous to infection. Furthermore, it does appear that higher doses are required to give a similar degree of inhibition to that observed in the infected cell system. Thus the effect of virus infection may be to enhance the antiviral effect of interferon *in vivo* rather than to be an absolute requirement.

The role of the virus in enhancing the effect of interferon treatment has been clarified by the finding that infection may be omitted if very small amounts of double-stranded polynucleotides are added to the cell-free system (Kerr *et al.*, 1974b). This suggests that it is double-stranded viral RNA made following infection, that "triggers" the latent antiviral state.

Fractionation of cell-free systems which display an interferon-mediated inhibition of translation indicate the existence of an inhibitor present in both the ribosomal and post-ribosomal supernatant fractions. The ribosome-bound inhibitor can be eluted by 0·5 M KCl and it has recently been reported that such an eluate from ribosomes from interferon-treated cells contains a polypeptide of molecular weight 48 000 which is not present in the corresponding fraction from untreated cells (Samuel and Joklik, 1974). This appears to be the first direct evidence for the existence of a new polypeptide in interferon-treated cells and which therefore may be equated with the hitherto hypothetical "antiviral protein".

One important property that one would expect of a well-behaved *in vitro* system displaying an interferon-mediated inhibition of translation is that of discrimination between viral and cellular messengers. Extracts from interferon-treated cells do appear to translate the synthetic message poly-(U) in all the studies noted above. In some cases, however, the translation of natural cellular messengers such as globin mRNA and total cellular mRNA, as well as viral mRNA, is inhibited (Falcoff *et al.*, 1973; Gupta *et al.*, 1973). Translation in these cell-free systems may not be functioning in precisely the same way as in the intact cell. In at least one cell-free system discrimination between cellular and viral mRNA translation has been reported (Samuel and Joklik, 1974). This system was prepared from interferon-treated but uninfected cells. Because of the possible role of very small amounts of double-stranded RNA in such a system, as noted above, and because exogeneous viral and cellular mRNA preparations might be contaminated by small amounts of double-stranded RNA, considerable caution must be exercised in the interpretation of such results at present.

To conclude a discussion on the mechanism of action of interferon attention should be drawn to the central puzzle which arises whether transcription or translation or both are inhibited. This is, how does the interferon-treated cell distinguish viral from cellular nucleic acids? It seems unlikely that interferon induces the synthesis of a distinct antiviral protein for each and every virus so there must exist a limited, possibly quite a small, number of characteristic nucleotide sequences which are not commonly present in cellular nucleic acids but one at least of which must be a component of nearly every viral genome. It is perhaps improbable that these viral nucleotide sequences are present only so that viruses should be sensitive to interferon; selective pressures would tend to work against that. If this is so then these sequences must serve some other purpose but what this may be is at present obscure.

4.3   ACTIVITIES OF INTERFERON OTHER THAN ANTIVIRAL

The biological activity that defines the substance known as interferon is, of course, the antiviral activity. In addition to this, however, a variety of other biological activities have been reported to be properties of interferon preparations. Since even in the most highly purified interferon preparations most of the protein is not interferon (see section 3.1) it remains uncertain whether or not these other activities are due to interferon itself or to impurities in the preparation. Certainly, the physiochemical properties and species specificities of the substances mediating these other activities are, in general, similar or identical to those of interferon itself. It is, however, conceivable that interferon is just one member of a class of secreted cellular proteins with similar physiochemical properties which convey information between cells. For this reason, and because nothing is known about the biochemical basis for these other various biological activities they will be described quite briefly.

Interferon has been found to be active against a number of nonviral infectious agents *in vivo* and *in vitro* (Merigan, 1973b). These are intracellular parasites of the classes chlamydiea (e.g. members of the trachoma-inclusion conjunctivitis group) and protozoa (e.g. *Toxoplasma gondii* and *Plasmodium berghei*). The organisms contain both DNA and RNA and have their own ribosomes.

There have been a number of reports that interferon preparations may inhibit cell division both *in vivo* and *in vitro*, including an extensive series of papers from Gresser and his co-workers (Gresser, 1972; Oxman, 1973). In general it appears that relatively large doses, compared to those required to demonstrate an antiviral effect, are necessary to show inhibition of cell division. Whether the anticellular activity is due to the same molecular species as the antiviral activity is not certain though highly purified preparations from a variety of sources display the same inhibitory effect (Gresser *et al.*, 1973). There is a suggestion, however, that the two activities may be physically separable (Borecky *et al.*, 1972; Matsuzawa and Kawade,

1974). The finding that sub-lines of cells which are resistant to the antiviral effect of interferon are also resistant to the inhibition of cell division would tend to support the notion that the two activities are mediated by the same molecular species (Gresser, 1972; Gresser *et al.*, 1974).

One interesting example of an effect of interferon on cell division *in vivo* is the report that large doses of interferon, when administered to mice two days before an antigen, will suppress the formation of the specific antibody producing spleen cells (Chester *et al.*, 1973). This might seem to be biologically disadvantageous but the dose of interferon required to suppress antibody production is ten- to one hundred-fold greater than that required to prevent lethal virus infection.

There are various reports that interferon treatment of uninfected cells may inhibit cellular macromolecular synthesis (Sonnabend and Friendman, 1973). For the reasons already discussed the status of such reports is uncertain. While the evidence for gross inhibition of macromolecular synthesis in uninfected cells is unconvincing, the possibility that limited and specific inhibitions or modifications occur cannot be disregarded. Indeed, it has been reported that messenger and transfer RNA from interferon-treated cells is larger than that from untreated cells (Levy and Riley, 1973). Moreover, the finding that the synthesis in uninfected cells of aryl hydrocarbon hydroxylase, an inducible cellular enzyme, is stimulated by pretreatment with interferon is both unexpected and interesting (Nebert and Friedman, 1973).

Priming activity is another type of activity that is induced by interferon treatment and which appears to be distinct from the antiviral activity. "Priming" describes the ability of interferon pretreatment of cells to enhance interferon yields following challenge with the inducing virus. For example, MM virus, a picornavirus, normally induces very little interferon in mouse L cells but when the cells are primed with a low dose of interferon the yields may be increased by a thousand-fold (Stewart *et al.*, 1971b). It might be thought that the effect of the primary dose of interferon was to inhibit some function of the inducing virus that blocked interferon synthesis. However, induction of interferon by poly(I).poly(C) may also be primed to some extent by interferon pretreatment and this suggests that priming enhances the sensitivity of the cells to the inducers in some manner not directly related to the antiviral activity.

Pretreatment of cells with interferon prior to induction does not always result in priming. Reduction in interferon yields may also be observed (Youngner and Hallum, 1969). This blocking activity has not been separated from the antiviral activity on extensive purification (Golgher and Paucker, 1973). There is some suggestion that pretreatment with low doses may enhance subsequent production whereas pretreatment with higher doses may hinder it (Friedman, 1966) but it is not clear that all findings may be explained in this way.

Another effect of interferon preparations on cells is to increase their susceptibility to the toxicity of poly(I).poly(C). Concentrations of poly-(I).poly(C) that produce no detectable toxicity in mouse L cells produce marked toxicity in L cells treated with interferon (Stewart *et al.*, 1972b). This enhanced susceptibility appears to be specific for double-stranded polynucleotides and not for other toxic materials (Stewart *et al.*, 1973a). The activity which enhances this toxicity co-purifies with the antiviral activity in interferon preparations (Stewart *et al.*, 1973b).

Other nonantiviral activities of interferon preparations that have been reported include enhancement of *in vitro* phagocytosis by mouse peritoneal phagocytes (Huang *et al.*, 1971), enhancement of the specific cytotoxicity of sensitized lymphocytes (Lindahl *et al.*, 1972), and inhibition of DNA synthesis induced in lymphocytes by nonviral stimuli (Lindahl-Magnusson *et al.*, 1972).

5 Interferon in animals and man

5.1 BIOLOGICAL ROLE OF INTERFERON

The very existence and properties of interferon obviously implies that it has a role in the defence of the organism against infection by viruses. Evidence bearing on the precise part that the interferon mechanism plays is largely circumstantial. The subject has recently been reviewed (Baron, 1973; Merigan, 1974) and only the main points will be mentioned here.

Interferon is only one of a number of host defence mechanism operating during virus infection. Others include neutralizing antibody, cellular immunity, local inflammation and generalized fever. Interferon has a broad antiviral effect and begins to operate within hours of infection. In contrast the immune system is virus specific and takes several days before it is functional. This would suggest that the interferon mechanism is the first line of defence against viral infection. At the site of initial virus infection the release of interferon from infected cells will protect adjacent cells and thus limit the spread of infection. Interferon appears in the serum within a few hours of the onset of viraemia. Experiments using passive transfer of interferon indicate that circulating interferon can both reduce the viraemia and protect target organs against infection with virus from the blood stream.

In addition to its role in the initial defence against infection interferon is also considered to play a part in recovery from a fully established infection (Baron, 1973). Thus it has been found that virus titres in infected tissues start to fall shortly after interferon is first detected in the tissue. For example, interferon in the vesicles of patients with a disseminated herpes zoster infection invariably reaches its maximum titre 48 hours prior to cessation of dissemination of the virus (Stevens, and Merigan, 1972).

When an animal is treated with a series of doses of an inducer at relatively short intervals the yield of interferon decreases with each successive stimulus. This phenomenon is known as hyporeactivity or refractiveness (see section 2.4). It is not obvious why this is the case, or, for that matter, why the interferon system is normally in a repressed state since it might be supposed that constant activity of the antiviral system or, at least, a readily repeatable inducibility would have some selective advantage. These aspects of the biological role of interferon have yet to be elucidated.

5.2   INTERFERON AND INTERFERON INDUCERS IN ANIMALS

The possibility that interferon and interferon inducers can be applied to medicine has prompted a large number of investigations of animal models. We will survey the field quite briefly since an extensive review has recently been published (Finter, 1973c). When interferon itself has been used it has to be remembered that in most studies crude or, at least, partially purified preparations have been used and thus some of the effects observed *in vivo* may have been due to contaminants. With inducers results may be more difficult to interpret since these have a variety of effects in animals in addition to their interferon-inducing ability (see below).

Our knowledge of the pharmacology and metabolic fate of interferon is fragmentory (Ho, 1973b). When administrated intravenously its concentration falls rapidly with a half-life of 20 minutes or less. Usually less than 10 per cent of the inoculum is recovered in the urine and the fate of the rest is unknown. When administered intramuscularly or subcutaneously a stable level of cirulatory interferon may be maintained for 12 hours or more (Cantell and Pyhälä, 1973). Little is known of the detailed distribution of systemically administered interferon. It appears to spread quite widely in the body but there seem to be some anatomical barriers to free diffusion. Thus the placenta acts as a barrier to interferon in the maternal circulation reaching the foetus (Ho *et al.*, 1967), although, interestingly, interferon can pass from lactating female mice to their newborn offspring via the milk (Schafer *et al.*, 1972).

Most animal studies of the protective effect of interferon have used the mouse. High titre mouse interferon is readily prepared from different sources and can be tested in a number of convenient experimental systemic infections. In general, a given amount of interferon is more effective against smaller rather than larger doses of virus, as expected. Interferon is most effective when given prior to infection. In a number of cases a protective effect has been demonstrated when interferon has been administered during a limited period after infection, especially when a relatively large dose has been used (Finter, 1967). Continual administration of interferon during the course of an experimental infection has been shown to be beneficial in some cases.

In addition to the experimental systemic infections mentioned above, interferon has also been shown to display some protective action against local infections. This is the case for vaccinia infection of the rabbit eye (Cantell and Tommila, 1960) and for influenza infection of the mouse respiratory tract (Finter, 1970).

The interferon inducers that have been most commonly used in animal experiments have been the double-stranded polynucleotides and preparations of fungal viruses containing this material. Microgram amounts of double-stranded polynucleotide injected intravenously lead to high titres of interferon in the blood of mice and other rodents within a few hours (Field et al., 1967a). Poly(I).poly(C) treatment has been shown to protect mice against a range of systemic virus infections (Finter, 1973c). Poly(I).poly(C) has also been shown to induce interferon synthesis when applied locally to the rabbit eye (Weissenbacher et al., 1970) and protection against herpes virus infection has been demonstrated (Park and Baron, 1968).

In systemic infections the protective effect of poly(I).poly(C) tends to be proportional to the dose of the inducer, at least up to a certain level, and inversely proportional to the dose of virus inoculum. The duration of protection of a single dose commonly lasts a number of days. Poly(I).poly(C) is most effective when administered before infection but a number of studies have shown significant protective effect when administration commenced after infection.

Although double-stranded polynucleotides are potent interferon inducers it cannot be assumed that the protective effect exerted in animals necessarily functions through this mechanism. Double-stranded polynucleotides may produce a wide variety of effects when administered to animals including enhancement of cell-mediated immunity, adjuvant activity and pyrogenic activity (Finter, 1973a). Clearly some of these other effects may contribute to the protective function.

There has been much recent interest in low molecular weight interferon inducers such as tilorone hydrochloride (section 2.1). Oral administration to mice results in the appearance of interferon in the serum (Mayer and Krueger, 1970) and protection against a variety of systemic virus infections. The dose used for protection was about one quarter of the LD_{50} and it appears that the drug is too toxic for use in medicine.

Finter (1973c, 1973d) has compared the relative advantages and disadvantages of interferon and inducers as potential antiviral drugs. Interferon itself appears to be nontoxic, is not antigenic in the homologous species and can be administered repeatedly without diminution of effect. On the other hand, the maximum antiviral effect is produced quite quickly and there may be problems producing sufficient amounts of interferon for therapeutic use. In contrast inducers are easier and cheaper to prepare and because they can lead to the formation of large amounts of interferon may have a prolonged antiviral effect. However, they all appear to be toxic at doses that are too close for comfort to the therapeutic doses and the phenomenon of hyperreactivity limits the frequency with which repeated doses may be given.

5.3   INTERFERON AND TUMOUR VIRUSES

Some viruses are known to be oncogenic; that is, they cause tumours in animals. Since interferon has a broad spectrum antiviral activity the possibility arises that it may have a protective effect against tumour formation by such viruses or even a therapeutic use against established tumours of viral or other origin. Only the most salient features of the extensive literature on this topic will be considered here. Comprehensive discussions may be found elsewhere (Oxman, 1973; Gresser, 1972).

Tumour viruses are able to induce tumours in appropriate host animals or to "transform" normal cells into tumour cells *in vitro*. A number of DNA and RNA viruses have this capacity. In the case of the DNA tumour viruses one may distinguish between essentially two types of virus–cell interaction. Infection of "permissive" cells gives rise to a cycle of productive infection in which progeny virus is liberated, while infection of "nonpermissive" cells does not yield progeny virus but instead a proportion of the cells may be transformed. For RNA tumour viruses, an infected cell is transformed and also liberates progeny virus. Transformation appears, in general, to involve the integration of part or all of a DNA virus genome (or a DNA copy of a RNA virus genome) into the cellular DNA with the subsequent expression of some of the viral genes. One result of this is that the morphology and growth behaviour of the cells is altered. Commonly they grow to higher densities and in a less regulated manner than normal cells.

In general, tumour viruses are indifferent inducers of interferon. This is true for both RNA and DNA viruses and, in the latter case, for both permissive and nonpermissive infections.

Tumour viruses vary in their sensitivity to interferon. The ability of RNA tumour viruses such as the avian or murine sarcoma viruses to form foci of transformed cells *in vitro* is inhibited by pretreatment of the cells with interferon. Focus formation is the result of multiple cycles of virus replication which lead to the infection and transformation of an increasing number of cells. Thus inhibition of focus formation probably reflects, to a large extent, inhibition of the replication of the virus itself. However, replication of RNA tumour viruses in tissue culture may be very sensitive to environmental factors and so it is particularly important to rule out cytotoxic or similar noninterferon effects of a preparation before concluding that a particular virus is sensitive to interferon.

The oncogenic DNA viruses vary widely in their sensitivity to interferon. Thus while polyoma virus is relatively resistant, SV40, a rather similar papovavirus, is quite sensitive (Oxman and Takemoto, 1970). Both lytic infection of permissive monkey cells by SV40 and transformation of non-permissive mouse cells are sensitive to monkey (and human) or mouse interferons respectively (Todaro and Baron, 1965; Oxman and Black, 1966). The adenoviruses appear to be fairly insensitive to interferon, at least in the cells that have been tested. Differences in oncogenicity of the various adenovirus types seem not to be related to their interferon sensitivity.

Pretreatment with interferon can inhibit tumour formation in animals following infection with certain RNA tumour viruses. This is the case for Rous sarcoma virus in chickens and the Friend and Rauscher leukemia viruses in mice. In the case of the murine viruses, interferon slowed the development of the disease even when treatment was not started until a week or more after the time of virus inoculation (Wheelock and Larke, 1968; Gresser, 1972). These beneficial effects of interferon *in vivo* are not unexpected since the viruses are known to be sensitive to interferon *in vitro* and tumour formation involves continuing virus replication and infection of previously uninvolved cells. On the other hand, it does not necessarily follow that the effects observed *in vivo* are necessarily due to interferon. The dominant role of the immune response in determining the outcome of tumour virus infections must be considered in all such experiments (Oxman, 1973). Small effects of interferon on host immunity resulting for example from the inhibition of an immunosuppressive passenger virus may indirectly inhibit the growth of a tumour and give an impression of a direct antiviral effect. Furthermore crude and partially purified interferon preparations may contain contaminants which enhance the host's immune defences.

There have been few studies of the effects of interferon on tumour formation in animals by DNA viruses, probably because the animal of choice for *in vivo* oncogenesis is the hamster and hamster interferon is difficult to prepare.

The use of interferon inducers to protect animals against infection with oncogenic viruses has obvious attractions and numerous such studies have been reported. For example, treatment of mice with poly(I).poly(C) before and during infection with a murine sarcoma virus reduced the incidence of tumour formation (Sarma *et al.*, 1969). However, the protective effect of poly(I).poly(C) on murine leukemia virus infection is more equivocal; beneficial or adverse effects may result depending on the dose and schedule of administration and the nature and time of the observations made (Larson *et al.*, 1969). Statolon, another interferon inducer, has been demonstrated to protect mice against infection with a murine leukemia virus (Wheelock *et al.*, 1971).

Although these interferon inducers will protect against infection with oncogenic viruses *in vivo* it seems more likely that they do so by enhancing the animal's immune response than by stimulating interferon synthesis. One piece of evidence in support of this view is that other effective inducers of interferon *in vivo*, such as Newcastle Disease virus, do not inhibit virus-induced leukemia in mice (Wheelock, 1966). Nevertheless, the induced interferon may play a secondary role, possibly by inhibiting the transient immunosuppression that is known to occur following infection with certain murine leukemia viruses and thereby allowing the enhanced host immune response to give prolonged protection.

Somewhat in contrast to the situation with RNA tumour viruses, interferon inducers seem to have little effect upon tumour formation by DNA tumour viruses. If their main effect was exerted via interferon induction as such this result would not be unexpected since, as noted already, DNA tumour viruses are relatively insensitive to interferon. If, however, the inducers were to act mainly on the host's immune system, as appears to be the case for the RNA tumour viruses, a greater protective effect might be anticipated. Possible explanations for the apparent anomaly include the following (Oxman, 1973). First, continuing virus replication is important in tumour progression in the case of RNA oncogenic viruses but not for the DNA tumour viruses; enhancement of virus neutralizing antibody may contribute to protection by inducers against the former class of tumours. Second, cells of tumours caused by RNA viruses, where progeny virions are continuously budding through the cellular membranes, may be more susceptible to the host's immune defences than those of DNA virus-induced tumours, where virus is not liberated. Third, a number of the murine RNA leukemia viruses suppress the immune response of the infected animal and in this situation the effect of an enhancer of this response may be more evident than in the case of a DNA tumour where immuno-suppression probably does not occur. Finally, most studies with RNA tumour viruses have employed mice while those with DNA tumour viruses more often use hamsters; the different effects of interferon inducers may simply reflect differences in the defence mechanism of these two animal species.

If, as is generally supposed, the altered properties of cells transformed by tumour viruses require the continued expression of one or more viral genes, then the possibility arises that interferon might act on such tumour cells to inhibit these viral functions and thereby cause the behaviour of the transformed cells to revert to normal. Such a result would have obvious implications for cancer therapy. However, in what is the clearest available example of an experiment of this type, the desired result was not obtained. Mouse cells transformed by SV40 express the viral T antigen and, while in a lytic infection this expression is quite sensitive to interferon, in transformed cells it is entirely insensitive (Oxman et al., 1967a). In the case of mouse cells transformed by a murine sarcoma virus, again viral antigens continued to be expressed during prolonged interferon treatment though, interestingly, reversion of some of the characteristics of the transformed cell phenotype were observed (Chaney and Vignal, 1970); the interpretation of this latter finding is not straightforward, however (Oxman, 1973).

Naturally, the effect of interferon and interferon inducers on transplantable tumours in animals has been investigated. For example, daily treatment with interferon following inoculation of mice with various ascites tumour cells has been reported to prolong markedly survival time (Gresser et al., 1969) although it is not clear that this effect was due to the antiviral activity of interferon (Oxman, 1973). In contrast a single dose of interferon has been reported to *enhance* the growth of a virus-induced sarcoma virus in mice (Gazdar et al., 1973). This may be due to suppression of the immune response of the treated animal (Chester et al., 1973).

Prolonged treatment with poly(I).poly(C) has been shown to inhibit the growth of a variety of transplantable mouse tumours including some which were originally spontaneous or were induced by chemical carcinogens (Levy et al., 1969). For reasons already discussed it seems unlikely that poly(I).poly(C) acts predominantly by inducing interferon synthesis. In contrast, however, a single dose of this inducer can enhance tumour growth (Gazdar, 1972).

In concluding this section it is worth emphasizing that while interferon preparations have been reported to inhibit transformation or tumour formation in a number of experimental systems the role of the antiviral activity of interferon is unclear. The position will only be clarified when highly purified interferon preparations can be used. It seems quite likely, however, that the interferon system has a certain role to play in the host's defences against viral neoplasia. Thus in view of the apparently negligible toxicity of interferon preparations, especially when contrasted with other modes of cancer chemotherapy, and despite the failure to demonstrate a clear viral aetiology in human, as opposed to animal, cancers, the use of highly purified human interferon in controlled trials in patients with cancer seems to be warranted.

5.4 INTERFERON AND INTERFERON INDUCERS IN MAN

The long-term aim of much of the work on the interferon system has been to develop therapy or prophylaxis of virus diseases in man. However, there have been only a few significant studies to date in which man has been the subject. These will now be reviewed quite briefly. A more extensive account of this topic is available (Finter, 1973d).

To put the problem of antiviral therapy into perspective it is necessary to emphasize the obvious fact that many serious human virus diseases are successfully controlled by immunization. There are, however, a number of situations when this is not the case. If the viral agent has not been isolated and grown *in vitro*, as in the case of viral hepatitis, then a vaccine cannot be prepared. Where the antigenic character of a virus may change rapidly, as in the case of influenza, there may be too little time to prepare a vaccine to ward off a major epidemic. Vaccine production is not practicable in the case of the common upper respiratory tract infections (the common cold) since the number of potential causative viruses is too large. Where a virus disease is serious yet uncommon it may not be desirable to vaccinate the whole population. Smallpox, rabies and the less common arboviruses fall into this category. Antiviral chemotherapy would be desirable in these situations as well as for immunosuppressed patients, where for example, latent herpes infections may become very serious, and in the relatively rare cases of viral encephalitis.

There are three general obstacles to antiviral chemotherapy (Fenner and White, 1970). First, there is the intimate relationship of viral metabolism to that of its host. Second, virus production is commonly, though not invariably, well advanced by the time symptoms become evident. Therapy may, nevertheless, speed recovery. Third, there is the danger that drug-resistant mutants may arise. The interferon mechanism compares favourably with conventional therapeutic agents in these respects. Evidently, it does distinguish viral functions in the intracellular milieu without general toxic effect on the organism. Less obviously, interferon-resistant mutants do not appear to arise either in nature or in the laboratory. This is surprising and the reason is unclear. The problem of late onset of symptoms in relation to the extent of virus multiplication remains but the broad spectrum of action of interferon is advantageous since precise early diagnosis is less important.

Quantitatively, if not qualitatively, the viral infections of the upper respiratory tract stand out as the current most serious problem of human virus disease. It seems likely that any widespread form of therapy or prophylaxis of the contacts of an infected subject will have to be self-administered. Clearly this requires a very low level of toxicity and undesirable side-effects. Here, interferon may well compare favourably with conventional antiviral drugs.

The difficulty of obtaining sufficient quantities of human interferon has severely limited human trials with interferon itself. Recently it has been demonstrated that a total of 14 million units of partially purified human leucocyte interferon administered intranasally in 39 doses both before and for 3 days after infection, were of benefit in experimental rhinovirus infection of volunteers (Merigan et al., 1973). The frequency of severe symptoms and of virus-shedding and the level of antibody response were all significantly reduced in the treated group compared with the control group. Where a lower dose of interferon was used (800 000 units) with an influenza virus challenge only a small delay in incubation period was observed. Russian workers have reported field trials in which relatively low doses of human interferon were claimed to give significant protection in a naturally occurring influenza epidemic (Solov'ev, 1969). However, the significance of these results is uncertain (Finter, 1973d; Jordan et al., 1973). Human interferon has been administered to cancer patients for prolonged periods with no serious toxic effect, though no beneficial effect either (Strander et al., 1973).

There has been one study of the effect of intranasal administration of poly(I).poly(C) on experimental infection of volunteers with rhinovirus and influenza virus (Hill et al., 1972). Despite the use of high local concentrations of the inducer (0.1 mg ml^{-1}) only a small reduction in symptoms was seen and decreased virus shedding was found in only one out of three trials. This may be because only very low levels of nasal interferon were detectable in the treated volunteers. On the other hand no detectable toxic effects of the polynucleotide were observed. Poly(I).poly(C) has been injected intravenously into patients with advanced cancer (Field et al., 1971). Fourteen out of 20 subjects responded by producing low titres of serum interferon. The only consistent clinical manifestation was a febrile response. In animals, particularly in dogs, poly(I).poly(C) is considerably more toxic (Hilleman, 1970). It is not clear at present whether there is a safe margin between the effective and toxic doses of double-stranded polynucleotides for man and in view of their known animal toxicity it seems unlikely that any of them will be licenced for human use. Veterinary use may be possible, however.

One of the low molecular weight interferon inducers, a substituted propanediamine (Hoffman et al., 1973) appears to be relatively nontoxic in man and there is one recent report of a study in volunteers in which significant protection against a rhinovirus challenge was claimed (Panusarn et al., 1974). A general problem with interferon inducers is that of hyporeactivity where repeated doses result in a reduced response (see section

2.4). On the other hand the use of human interferon itself does not appear to raise problems of toxicity or hyporeactivity; the present difficulty is one of supply. The main current source of human interferon is from human leucocytes infected with a paramyxovirus (Falcoff *et al.*, 1966; Strander *et al.*, 1973). The human dose of 14 million units referred to above derived from thirty to fifty 500 ml blood transfusion donations (Merigan *et al.*, 1973). A further problem with leucocytes is the possibility of contamination with hepatitis virus although precautions against this may be taken (Andrews *et al.*, 1970). Continuous human cell lines which are good interferon producers clearly are needed. In the long run it may be possible to make or select cell variants which synthesize interferon constitutively, but our ability to manipulate the mammalian genome does not yet permit this.

Improvements in purification methods, particularly the use of affinity chromatography (section 3.1), should readily allow a sufficient degree of purification of human interferon for clinical use. Purification of mouse interferon may now be approaching the point where a single, homogeneous component can be obtained. Work on human interferon has lagged some way behind but one may anticipate that it will be purified to homogeneity in due course. When sufficient pure interferon is obtained it should be possible to determine the amino acid sequence and then the chemical synthesis of the protein could be contemplated. While such a synthesis would be a formidable undertaking, interferon made in this way might be more economic than that derived from cell culture. If the specific activity of pure interferon were of the order of 10^9 units per mg protein (see section 3.1) and the amount required for a course of treatment were about 10^8 units, then one gram of synthetic interferon would provide material for 10 000 patients. In their laboratory-scale synthesis of ribonuclease Gutte and Merrifield (1971) prepared 130 mg of the purified protein. Amino acid sequence determination and chemical synthesis would be expedited, of course, if human interferon were comprised of subunits of 12 000 molecular weight or smaller, as has been proposed (see section 3.2).

Other means of exploiting the interferon mechanism for human therapy may arise from a better understanding of the biochemistry of interferon induction and action. An important question on the subject of induction is whether toxicity and interferon-inducing ability are necessarily correlated. If they are not inducers may yet be of practical importance. Present data suggests, however, that toxicity and antiviral activity are closely correlated (Black *et al.*, 1973).

In the case of interferon action, it is possible that a detailed understanding of the molecular mechanisms involved, in particular how viral nucleic acids are distinguished from cellular, will eventually lead to the synthesis of drugs which will mimic the action of the intracellular inhibitor. Conceivably these may be of relatively low molecular weight.

When interferon was first discovered there was considerable hope that it could quickly be applied to the treatment of human virus infection. It did not seem too optimistic to expect that it would be to virus diseases what penicillin had been to bacterial infections. This early vision gradually faded as the logistic problems of producing human interferon on a sufficient scale became apparent. Ten years after its discovery the notion that interferon might be useful therapeutically received a considerable stimulus from the discovery of the potent inducing ability of double-stranded polynucleotides. Again the initial enthusiasm has waned as the close correlation between interferon-inducing ability and toxicity has become evident.

Although progress in exploiting the interferon phenomenon has been slow, advances in conventional chemotherapy of virus infection have been equally undramatic. Despite the difficulties, the wide spectrum of antiviral activity together with the absence of toxicity suggests that the interferon mechanism remains the most plausible approach to the therapy of virus diseases.

Acknowledgements

This review was written while the author was visiting the Virus Research Unit of the Children's Hospital Medical Center, Boston, Massachussetts. The hospitality of Drs J. F. Enders and M. N. Oxman is gratefully acknowledged.

References

Andrews, R. D., Appleyard, G., Beale, A. J., Bucknall, R. A., Cantell, K., Clark, M., Clements, E. M. B., Draper, C. C., Fantes, K. H., Finter, N. B., Nevanlinna, H., Perkins, F. T., Tyrrell, D. A. J. and Whittaker, A. (1970). *Annals of the New York Academy of Science*, **173**, 770.

Anfinsen, C. B., Bose, S., Corley, L. and Gurari-Rotman, D. (1974). *Proceedings of the National Academy of Sciences, USA*, **71**, 3139.

Ankel, H., Chany, C., Galliot, B., Chevalier, M. J., and Robert, M. (1973). *Proceedings of the National Academy of Sciences, USA*, **70**, 2360.

Atkins, G. J., Johnston, M. D., Westmacott, L. M. and Burke, D. C. (1974). *Journal of General Virology*, **25**, 381.

Bakay, M. and Burke, D. C. (1972). *Journal of General Virology* **16**, 399.

Baltimore, D. (1969). *In* "Biochemistry of Viruses" (Ed. H. B. Levy), p. 101. Marcel Dekker, New York.

Baron, S. (1973). *In* "Interferons and Interferon Inducers" (Ed. N. B. Finter), p. 267. North-Holland, Amsterdam and London.

Baron, S. and Buckler, C. E. (1963). *Science*, **141**, 1061.

Baron, S., Buckler, C. E., Levy, H. B. and Friedman, R. M. (1967). *Proceedings of the Society for Experimental Biology and Medicine*, **125**, 1320.

Baron, S., Bogomolova, N. N., Billiau, A., Levy, H. B., Buckler, C. E., Stern, R. and Naylor, R. (1969). *Proceedings of the National Academy of Sciences, USA,* **64**, 67.

Bausek, G. H. and Merigan, T. C. (1969). *Virology,* **39**, 491.

Bean, W. J. and Simpson, R. W. (1973). *Virology,* **56**, 646.

Beers, R. F. and Braun, W. (eds) (1971). "Biological Effects of Polynucleotides". Springer-Verlag, New York, Heidelberg and Berlin.

Bialy, H. S. and Colby, C. (1972). *Journal of Virology,* **9**, 286.

Black, D. R., Eckstein, F., Hobbs, J. B., Sternbach, H. and Merigan, T. C. (1972). *Virology,* **48**, 537.

Black, D. R., Eckstein, F., De Clercq, E. and Merigan, T. C. (1973). *Antimicrobial Agents and Chemotherapy,* **3**, 198.

Borecky, L., Fuchsberger, N., Hájnická, V., Stanček, D. and Žemla, J. (1972). *Acta Virologica (Prague), English Edition,* **16**, 356.

Buckler, C. E., Baron, S. and Levy, H. (1966). *Science,* **152**, 80.

Bucknall, R. A. (1967). *Nature (London),* **216**, 1022.

Burgess, R. R., Travers, A. A., Dunn, J. J. and Bautz, E. K. F. (1969). *Nature (London),* **221**, 43.

Burke, D. C. (1973). *In* "Interferons and Interferon Inducers" (Ed. N. B. Finter), p. 107. North-Holland, Amsterdam and London.

Cantell, K. and Paucker, K. (1963). *Virology,* **10**, 81.

Cantell, K. and Pyhälä, L. (1973). *Journal of General Virology,* **20**, 97.

Cantell, K. and Tommila, V. (1960). *Lancet,* **ii**, 682.

Carter, W. A. (1970). *Proceedings of the National Academy of Sciences, USA,* **67**, 620.

Carter, W. A. and Levy, H. B. (1967). *Science,* **155**, 1254.

Carter, W. A., Pitha, P. M., Marshall, L. W., Tazawa, I., Tazawa, S. and Ts'O, P. O. P. (1972). *Journal of Molecular Biology,* **70**, 567.

Cassingena, R., Chany, C., Vignal, M., Suarez, H., Estrade, S. and Lazar, P. (1971). *Proceedings of the National Academy of Sciences USA,* **68**, 580.

Chandra, P., Zunino, F., Gaur, V. P., Zaccara, A., Wottersdorf, M., Luoni, G. and Götz, A. (1972). *FEBS Letter,* **28**, 5.

Chany, C. and Vignal, M. (1970). *Journal of General Virology,* **7**, 203.

Chany, C., Fournier, F. and Rousset, S. (1971). *Nature (London), New Biology,* **230**, 113.

Chany, C., Grégoire, A., Vignal, M., Lemaitre-Moncuit, J., Brown, P., Besançon, F., Suarez, H. and Cassingena, R. (1973). *Proceedings of the National Academy of Sciences, USA,* **70**, 557.

Chany, C., Ankel, H., Galliot, B., Chevalier, M. J. and Gregoire, A. (1974). Proceedings of the Society for Experimental Biology and Medicine, **147**, 293.

Chester, T. J., Paucker, K. and Merigan, T. C. (1973). *Nature (London),* **246**, 92.

Clavell, L. A. and Bratt, M. A. (1971). *Journal of Virology,* **8**, 500.

Colby, C. (1971). *Progress in Nucleic Acid Research and Molecular Biology,* **11**, 1.

Colby, C. and Chamberlin, M. J. (1969). *Proceedings of the National Academy of Sciences, USA,* **63**, 160.

Colby, C. and Duesberg, P. H. (1969). *Nature (London),* **222**, 940.

Colby, C. and Morgan, M. J. (1971). *Annual Reviews of Microbiology,* **25**, 333.

Colby, C., Jurale, C. and Kates, J. R. (1971). *Journal of Virology,* **7**, 71.

De Clercq, E. and De Somer, P. (1972). *Journal of Virology,* **9**, 721.

De Clercq, E. and Janik, B. (1973). *Biochimica et Biophysica Acta*, **324**, 50.

De Clercq, E. and Merigan, T. C. (1969). *Nature (London)*, **222**, 1148.

De Clercq, E. and Merigan, T. C. (1970). *Annual Reviews of Medicine*, **21**, 17.

De Clercq, E. and Merigan, T. C. (1971). *Journal of Infectious Diseases*, **123**, 190.

De Clercq, E. and Stewart, W. E. (1974). *Journal of General Virology*, **24**, 201.

De Clercq, E., Eckstein, F. and Merigan, T. C. (1969), *Science*, **165**, 1137.

De Clercq, E., Eckstein, F. and Merigan, T. C. (1970). *Annals of the New York Academy of Sciences*, **173**, 444.

De Clercq, E., Wells, R. D., Grant, R. C. and Merigan, T. C. (1971). *Journal of Molecular Biology*, **56**, 83.

De Clercq, E., Wells, R. D. and Merigan, T. C. (1972a). *Virology*, **47**, 405.

De Clercq, E., Zmudzka, B. and Shugar, D. (1972b). *FEBS Letter*, **24**, 137.

De Clercq, E., Torrence, P. F. and Witkop, B. (1974). *Proceedings of the National Academy of Sciences, USA*, **71**, 182.

De Maeyer, E. and De Maeyer-Guignard, J. (1969). *Journal of Virology*, **3**, 506.

De Maeyer, E., De Maeyer-Guignard, J. and Jullien, P. (1969). *Proceedings of the Society for Experimental Biology and Medicine*, **131**, 36.

De Maeyer-Guignard, J., De Maeyer, E. and Jullien, P. (1969). *Proceedings of the National Academy of Sciences, USA*, **63**, 732.

De Maeyer-Guignard, J., De Maeyer, E. and Montagnier, L. (1972). *Proceedings of the National Academy of Sciences, USA*, **69**, 1203.

Desmyter, J., Rawls, W. E. and Melnick, J. L. (1968). *Proceedings of the National Academy of Sciences, USA*, **59**, 69.

Dianzani, F., Cantagalli, P., Gagnoni, S. and Rita, G. (1968). *Proceedings of the Society for Experimental Biology and Medicine*, **128**, 708.

Dianzani, F., Buckler, C. E. and Baron, S. (1969). *Proceedings of the Society for Experimental Biology and Medicine*, **130**, 519.

Dorner, F., Scriba, M. and Weil, R. (1973). *Proceedings of the National Academy of Sciences, USA*, **70**, 1981.

Epstein, L. B., Cline, M. J. and Merigan, T. C. (1971a). *Cell Immunology*, **2**, 602.

Epstein, L. B., Cline, M. J. and Merigan, T. C. (1971b). *Journal of Clinical Investigation*, **50**, 744.

Epstein, L. B., Stevens, D. A. and Merigan, T. C. (1972). *Proceedings of the National Academy of Sciences, USA*, **69**, 2632.

Esteban, M. and Metz, D. H. (1973). *Journal of General Virology*, **20**, 111.

Falcoff, E., Falcoff, R., Fournier, F., Chany, C. and Galliot, B. (1966). *Annales d'l'Institut Pasteur*, **111**, 562.

Falcoff, E., Falcoff, R., Lebleu, B. and Revel, M. (1972). *Nature (London), New Biology*, **240**, 145.

Falcoff, E., Falcoff, R., Lebleu, B. and Revel, M. (1973). *Journal of Virology*, **12**, 421.

Fantes, K. H. (1967). *Journal of General Virology*, **1**, 257.

Fantes, K. H. (1969). *Science*, **163**, 1198.

Fantes, K. H. (1970). *Annals of the New York Academy of Science*, **173**, 118.

Fantes, K. H. (1973). *In* "Interferons and Interferon Inducers" (Ed. N. B. Finter), p. 171. North-Holland, Amsterdam and London.

Fantes, K. H. and Furminger, I. G. S. (1967). *Nature*, **216**, 71.

Fenner, F. and White, D. O. (1970). "Medical Virology". Academic Press, New York and London.

Field, A. K., Tytell, A. A., Lampson, G. P. and Hilleman, M. R. (1967a). *Proceedings of the National Academy of Sciences, USA*, **58**, 1004.

Field, A. K., Lampson, G. P., Tytell, A. A., Nemes, M. M. and Hilleman, M. R. (1967b). *Proceedings of the National Academy of Sciences, USA*, **58**, 2102.

Field, A. K., Young, C. W., Krakoff, I. H., Tytell, A. A., Lampson, G. P., Nemes, M. M. and Hilleman, M. R. (1971). *Proceedings of the Society for Experimental Biology and Medicine*, **136**, 1180.

Field, A. K., Lampson, G. P., Tytell, A. A. and Hilleman, M. R. (1972). *Proceedings of the Society for Experimental Biology and Medicine*, **141**, 440.

Finter, N. B. (1967). *Journal of General Virology*, **1**, 395.

Finter, N. B. (1970). *Annals of the New York Academy of Sciences*, **173**, 131.

Finter, N. B. (1973a). "Interferon and Interferon Inducers." North-Holland, Amsterdam and London.

Finter, N. B. (1973b). *In* "Interferons and Interferon Inducers" (Ed. N. B. Finter), p. 135. North-Holland, Amsterdam and London.

Finter, N. B. (1973c). *In* "Interferons and Interferon Inducers" (Ed. N. B. Finter), p. 295, North-Holland, Amsterdam and London.

Finter, N. B. (1973d). *In* "Interferons and Interferon Inducers" (Ed. N. B. Finter), p. 363. North-Holland, Amsterdam and London.

Friedman, R. M. (1966). *Journal of Immunology*, **96**, 872.

Friedman, R. M. (1967). *Science*, **156**, 1760.

Friedman, R. M. (1968). *Journal of Virology*, **2**, 1081.

Friedman, R. M. (1970). *Journal of General Physiology*, **56**, 149S.

Friedman, R. M., Fantes, K. H., Levy, H. B. and Carter, W. B. (1967). *Journal of Virology*, **1**, 1168.

Friedman, R. M., Metz, D. H., Esteban, R. M., Tovell, D. R., Ball, L. A. and Kerr, I. M. (1972). *Journal of Virology*, **10**, 1184.

Gauntt, C. J. and Lockart, R. Z. (1968). *Journal of Virology*, **2**, 567.

Gazdar, A. F. (1972). *Journal of the National Cancer Institute*, **49**, 1435.

Gazdar, A. F., Sims, H., Spahn, G. J. and Baron, S. (1973). *Nature (London), New Biology*, **245**, 77.

Gifford, G. E. and Koch, A. L. (1969). *Journal of Theoretical Biology*, **22**, 271.

Golgher, R. R. and Paucker, K. (1973). *Proceedings of the Society for Experimental Biology and Medicine*, **142**, 167.

Green, J. A., Cooperband, S. R. and Kibrick, S. (1969), *Science*, **164**, 1415.

Gresser, I. (1972). *In* "Advances in Cancer Research" (Eds G. Klein and S. Weinhouse), vol. 16, p. 97. Academic Press, New York and London.

Gresser, I., Bourali, C., Levy, J. P., Fontaine-Brouty-Boyé, D. and Thomas, M. T. (1969). *Proceedings of the National Academy of Sciences, USA*, **63**, 51.

Gresser, I., Bandu, M.-T., Tovey, M., Bodo, G., Paucker, K. and Stewart, W. (1973). *Proceedings of the Society for Experimental Biology and Medicine*, **142**, 7.

Gresser, I., Bandu, M.-T. and Brouty-Boyé, D. (1974). *Journal of the National Cancer Institute*, **52**, 553.

Gupta, S. L., Sopori, M. L. and Lengyel, P. (1973). *Biochemical and Biophysical Research Communications*, **54**, 777.

Gupta, S. L., Graziadei, W. D., Weideli, H., Sopori, M. L. and Lengyel, P. (1974). *Virology*, **57**, 49.

Gutte, B. and Merrifield, R. B. (1971). *Journal of Biological Chemistry*, **246**, 1922.

Haase, A. T., Baron, S., Levy, H. and Kasel, J. A. (1969). *Journal of Virology*, **4**, 490.

Hallum, J. V. and Youngner, J. S. (1966). *Journal of Bacteriology*, **92**, 1047.

Hallum, J. V., Thacore, H. R. and Youngner, J. S. (1970). *Journal of Virology*, **6**, 156.

Heller, E. (1963). *Virology*, **21**, 652.

Hill, D. A., Baron, S., Perkins, J. C., Worthington, M., Van Kirk, J. E., Mills, J., Kapikian, A. Z. and Chanock, R. M. (1972). *Journal of the American Medical Association*, **219**, 1179.

Hilleman, M. R., (1970). *Journal of Infectious Diseases*, **121**, 196.

Ho, M. (1973a). *In* "Interferons and Interferon Inducers" (Ed. N. B. Finter), p. 29. North-Holland, Amsterdam and London.

Ho, M. (1973b). *In* "Interferons and Interferon Inducers" (Ed. N. B. Finter), p. 73. North-Holland, Amsterdam and London.

Ho, M. (1973c). *In* "Interferons and Interferon Inducers" (Ed. N. B. Finter), p. 241. North-Holland, Amsterdam and London.

Ho, M., Postic, B. and Ke, Y. H. (1967). *In* "Ciba Foundation Symposium on Interferon" (Eds G. E. W. Wolstenholme and M. O'Connor), p. 19. Churchill, London.

Hoffman, W. W., Korst, J. J., Niblack, J. F. and Cronin, T. H. (1973). *Antimicrobial Agents and Chemotherapy*, **3**, 498.

Huang, K.-Y., Donahoe, R. M., Gordon, F. B. and Dressler, H. R. (1971). *Infection and Immunity*, **4**, 581.

Isaacs, A. and Lindenmann, J. (1957). *Proceedings of the Royal Society (London) Ser. B.*, **147**, 258.

Jacob, F. and Monod, J. (1961). *Journal of Molecular Biology*, **3**, 318.

Joklik, W. K. and Merigan, T. C. (1966). *Proceedings of the National Academy of Sciences, USA*, **56**, 558.

Jordan, W. S., Hopps, H. E. and Merigan, T. C. (1973). *Journal of Infectious Diseases*, **128**, 261.

Jungwirth, C., Horak, I., Bodo, G., Lindner, J. and Schultze, B. (1972). *Virology*, **48**, 59.

Kerr, I. M. (1971). *Journal of Virology*, **7**, 448.

Kerr, I. M., Sonnabend, J. A. and Martin, E. M. (1970). *Journal of Virology*, **5**, 132.

Kerr, I. M., Friedman, R. F., Brown, R. E., Ball, L. A. and Brown, J. C. (1974a). *Journal of Virology*, **13**, 9.

Kerr, I. M., Brown, R. E. and Ball, L. A. (1974b). *Nature*, **250**, 57.

Kleinschmidt, W. J. (1972). *Annual Reviews of Biochemistry*, **41**, 517.

Kleinschmidt, W. J. and Ellis, L. F. (1967). *Nature (London)*, **215**, 649.

Kleinschmidt, W. J., Cline, J. C. and Murphy, E. B. (1964). *Proceedings of the National Academy of Sciences, USA*, **52**, 741.

Knight, Jr., E. (1974). *Biochemical and Biophysical Research Communications*, **56**, 860.

Krueger, R. F. and Mayer, G. D. (1970). *Science*, **169**, 1213.

Lai, M.-H. T. and Joklik, W. K. (1973). *Virology*, **51**, 191.

Lampson, G. P., Tytell, A. A., Field, A. K., Nemes, M. M. and Hilleman, M. R. (1967). *Proceedings of the National Academy of Sciences, USA*, **58**, 782.

Larson, V. M., Clark, W. R. and Hilleman, M. R. (1969). *Proceedings of the Society for Experimental Biology and Medicine*, **131**, 1002.

Levy, H. B. and Carter, W. A. (1968). *Journal of Molecular Biology*, **31**, 561.

Levy, H. B. and Riley, F. L. (1973). *Proceedings of the National Academy of Sciences, USA*, **70**, 3815.

Levy, H. B., Law, L. W. and Rabson, A. S. (1969). *Proceedings of the National Academy of Science, USA*, **62**, 357.

Levy-Koenig, R. E., Mundy, M. J. and Paucker, K. (1970a). *Journal of Immunology*, **104**, 785.

Levy-Koenig, R. E., Golgher, R. R. and Paucker, K. (1970b). *Journal of Immunology*, **104**, 791.

Lindhal, P., Leary, P. and Gresser, I. (1972). *Proceedings of the National Academy of Sciences, USA*, **69**, 721.

Lindahl-Magnusson, P., Leary, P. and Gresser, I. (1972). *Nature (London), New Biology*, **237**, 120.

Lockart, R. Z. (1973). *In* "Interferon and Interferon Inducers" (Ed. N. B. Finter), p. 11. North-Holland, Amsterdam and London.

Lockart, R. Z., Bayliss, N. L., Toy, S. T. and Yin, F. H. (1968). *Journal of Virology*, **2**, 962.

Lomniczi, N. B. and Burke, D. C. (1970). *Journal of General Virology*, **8**, 55.

Magee, N., Levine, S., Miller, O. V. and Hamilton, R. D. (1968). *Virology*, **35**, 505.

Manders, E. K., Tilles, J. G. and Huang, A. S. (1972). *Virology*, **49**, 573.

Marcus, P. I. and Salb, J. M. (1966). *Virology*, **30**, 502.

Marcus, P. I., Engelhart, D. L., Hunt, J. M. and Sekellick, M. J. (1971). *Science*, **174**, 593.

Marshall, L. W., Pitha, P. M. and Carter, W. A. (1972). *Virology*, **48**, 607.

Matsuzawa, T. and Kawade, Y. (1974). *Acta Virologia*, **18**, 383.

Mayer, G. D. and Krueger, R. F. (1970). *Science*, **169**, 1214.

Mecs, E., Sonnabend, J. A., Martin, E. M. and Fantes, K. H. (1967). *Journal of General Virology*, **1**, 25.

Merigan, T. C. (1973a). *In* "Interferon and Interferon Inducers" (Ed. N. B. Finter), p. 45. North-Holland, Amsterdam and London.

Merigan, T. C. (1973b). *In* "Interferon and Interferon Inducers" (Ed. N. B. Finter), p. 251. North-Holland, Amsterdam, London.

Merigan, T. C. (1974). *New England Journal of Medicine*, **290**, 323.

Merigan, T. C., Reed, S. E., Hall, T. S. and Tyrrell, D. A. J. (1973). *Lancet*, **i**, 563.

Metz, D. H. and Esteban, M. (1972). *Nature (London)*, **238**, 385.

Metz, D. H., Esteban, M. and Danielescu, G. (1975). *Journal of General Virology*. **27**, 197.

Mogensen, K. E. and Cantell, K. (1974). *Journal of General Virology*, **22**, 95.

Montagnier, L., Collandre, H., De Maeyer-Guignard, J. and De Maeyer, E. (1974). *Biochemical and Biophysical Research Communications*, **59**, 1031.

Nebert, D. W. and Friedman, R. M. (1973). *Journal of Virology*, **11**, 193.

Ng, M. N. and Vilček, J. (1972). *In* "Advances in Protein Chemistry" (Eds C. B. Anfinsen, J. T. Edsall and F. M. Richards). Academic Press, New York and London.

Niblack, J. F. and McCreary, M. B. (1971). *Nature (London), New Biology*, **233**, 52.

Ogburn, C. A., Berg, K. and Paucker, K. (1973). *Journal of Immunology*, **111**, 1206.

Oie, H. K., Gazdar, A. F., Buckler, C. E. and Baron, S. (1972). *Journal of General Virology*, **17**, 107.

Oxman, M. N. (1973). *In* "Interferon and Interferon Inducers" (Ed. N. B. Finter), p. 391. North-Holland, Amsterdam and London.

Oxman, M. N. and Black, P. H. (1966). *Proceedings of the National Academy of Sciences, USA*, **55**, 1133.

Oxman, M. N. and Levin, M. (1971). *Proceedings of the National Academy of Sciences, USA*, **68**, 299.

Oxman, M. N. and Takemoto, K. K. (1970). *In Colloque Nr 6, Institut National de la Santé et de la Recherche Médicale*, p. 429.

Oxman, M. N., Baron, S., Black, P. H., Takemoto, K. K., Habel, K. and Rowe W. P. (1967a). *Virology*, **32**, 122.

Oxman, M. N., Rowe, W. P. and Black, P. H. (1967b). *Proceedings of the National Academy of Sciences, USA*, **57**, 941.

Oxman, M. N., Levin, M. J. and Lewis, A. M. (1974). *Journal of Virology*, **13**, 32.

Palmiter, R. D. and Schimke, R. T. (1973). *Journal of Biological Chemistry*, **248**, 1502.

Panusarn, C., Stanley, E. D., Dirda, V., Rubenis, M. and Jackson, G. G. (1974). *New England Journal of Medicine*, **291**, 57.

Park, J. H. and Baron, S. (1968). *Science*, **162**, 811.

Paucker, K. and Boxaca, M. (1967). *Bacteriological Reviews*, **31**, 145.

Paucker, K., Berman, B. J., Golgher, R. R. and Staňcek, D. (1970). *Journal of Virology*, **5**, 145.

Pitha, P. M. and Carter, W. A. (1971a). *Nature (London), New Biology*, **234**, 105.

Pitha, P. M. and Carter, W. A. (1971b). *Virology*, **45**, 777.

Pitha, P. M. and Pitha, J. (1973). *Journal of General Virology*, **21**, 31.

Radke, K. L., Colby, C., Kates, J. R., Krider, H. M. and Prescott, D. M. (1974). *Journal of Virology*, **13**, 623.

Rang, H. P. (1971). *Nature (London)*, **231**, 91.

Repik, P., Flamand, A. and Bishop, D. H. L. (1974). *Journal of Virology*, **14**, 1169.

Riley, B. P. and Gifford, G. E. (1967). *Journal of General Microbiology*, **46**, 293.

Samuel, C. E. and Joklik, W. K. (1974). *Virology*, **58**, 476.

Sarma, P. S., Shui, G. Neubauer, R., Baron, S. and Huebner, R. J. (1969). *Proceedings of the National Academy of Sciences, USA*, **62**, 1046.

Schonne, E., Billiau, A. and De Somer, P. (1970). *In* "International Symposium on Standardisation of Interferon and Interferon Inducers" (Eds F. T. Perkins and R. H. Regamey), p. 61. Karger, Basel.

Shafer, T. W. and Lockart, R. Z. (1970). *Nature (London)*, **226**, 449.

Shafer, T. W., Lieberman, M., Cohen, M. and Came, P. E. (1972). *Science*, **176**, 1326.

Sheaff, E. T. and Stewart, R. B. (1969). *Canadian Journal of Microbiology*, **15**, 941.

Sheaff, E. T., Meager, A. and Burke, D. C. (1972). *Journal of General Virology*, **17**, 163.

Shope, R. E. (1948). *American Journal of Botany*, **35**, 803.

Sipe, J., De Maeyer-Guignard, J., Fauconnier, B. and De Maeyer, E. (1973). *Proceedings of the National Academy of Science, USA*, **70**, 1037.

Solov'ev, V. D. (1969). *Bulletin of the World Health Organization*, **41**, 683.

Sonnabend, J. A. and Friedman, R. M. (1973). *In* "Interferon and Interferon Inducers" (Ed. N. B. Finter), p. 201. North-Holland, Amsterdam and London.

Sonnabend, J. A., Martin, E. M., Mecs, E. and Fantes, K. H. (1967). *Journal of General Virology*, **1**, 41.

Sonnabend, J. A., Kerr, I. M. and Martin, E. M. (1970). *Journal of General Physiology*, **56**, 172S.

Stanček, D. and Paucker, K. (1971). *Applied Microbiology*, **21**, 1067.

Stewart, W. E. (1974). *Virology*, **61**, 80.

Stewart, W. E. and De Clercq, E. (1974). *Journal of General Virology*, **23**, 83.

Stewart, W. E., Scott, W. D. and Sulkin, S. E. (1969). *Journal of Virology*, **4**, 147.

Stewart, W. E., Gosser, L. B. and Lockart, R. Z. (1971a). *Journal of General Virology*, **13**, 35.

Stewart, W. E., Gosser, L. B. and Lockart, R. Z. (1971b). *Journal of Virology*, **7**, 792.

Stewart, W. E., De Clercq, E. and De Somer (1972a). *Journal of Virology*, **10**, 707.

Stewart, W. E., De Clercq, E., Billiau, A., Desmyter, J. and De Somer, P. (1972b). *Proceedings of the National Academy of Sciences, USA*, **69**, 1851.

Stewart, W. E., De Clercq, E. and De Somer, P. (1973a). *Journal of General Virology*, **18**, 237.

Stewart, W. E., De Clercq, E. De Somer, P., Berg, K., Ogburn, C. A. and Paucker, K. (1973b). *Nature (London), New Biology*, **246**, 141.

Strander, H. and Cantell, K. (1966). *Annales Medicinae Experimentalie et Biologiae Fenniae*, **44**, 265.

Strander, H., Cantell, K., Carlström, G. and Jacobsson, P. Å. (1973). *Journal of the National Cancer Institute*, **51**, 733.

Stevens, D. A. and Merigan, T. C. (1972). *Journal of Clinical Investigations*, **51**, 1170.

Stinebring, W. R. and Absher, M. (1970). *In* "Biological Effects of Polynucleotides" (Eds R. F. Beers and W. Braun), p. 249. Springer-Verlag, New York, Heidelberg, Berlin.

Talal, N. (1971). *Agents and Actions*, **2**, 45.

Tan, Y. H., Armstrong, J. A., Ke, Y. H. and Ho, M. (1970). *Proceedings of the National Academy of Sciences, USA*, **67**, 464.

Tan, Y. H., Tischfield, J. and Ruddle, F. H. (1973). *Journal of Experimental Medicine*, **134**, 317.

Tan, Y. H., Creagan, R. P. and Ruddle, F. H. (1974). *Proceedings of the National Academy of Sciences, USA*, **71**, 2251.

Taylor, J. (1964). *Biochemical Research Communications*, **14**, 447.

Taylor-Papadimitriou, J. and Kallos, J. (1973). *Nature (London), New Biology*, **245**, 143.

Todaro, G. J. and Baron, S. (1965). *Proceedings of the National Academy of Sciences, USA*, **54**, 752.

Tomkins, G. M., Gelehrter, T. D., Granner, D., Martin, D., Samuels, H. H. and Thompson, E. B. (1969). *Science*, **166**, 1474.

Tomkins, G. M., Levinson, B. B., Baxter, J. D. and Dethlefsen, L. (1972). *Nature (London), New Biology*, **239**, 9.

Torrence, P. F., Bobst, A. M., Waters, J. A. and Witkop, B. (1973). *Biochemistry*, **12**, 3962.

Tovey, M. G., Mathison, G. E. and Pirt, S. J. (1973). *Journal of General Virology*, **20**, 29.

Tytell, A. A., Lampson, G. P., Field, A. K. and Hilleman, M. R. (1967). *Proceedings of the National Academy of Sciences, USA*, **58**, 1719.

Uhlendorf, C. P., Zimmerman, E. M. and Baron, S. (1974). *Proceedings of the Society for Experimental Biology and Medicine*, **144**, 628.

Ustacelebi, S. and Williams, J. F. (1972). *Nature (London)*, **235**, 52.

Vilček, J. (1969). "Interferon". Virology Monographs, vol. 6. Springer-Verlag, Wien and New York.

Vilček, J. and Havell, E. A., (1973). *Proceedings of the National Academy of Sciences, USA*, **70**, 3909.

Vilček, J. and Ng, M. H. (1971). *Journal of Virology*, **7**, 588.

Wacker, A., Lodemann, E., Diederich, J., Mohrbutter, K. and Lauschke, U. (1972). *Archiv. für Gesamte Virusforshung*, **36**, 71.

Wagner, R. R. (1964). *Nature (London)*, **204**, 49.

Wagner, R. R. and Huang, A. S. (1965). *Proceedings of the National Academy of Sciences*, **54**, 1112.

Weissenbacher, M., Schachter, N., Galin, M. A. and Baron, S. (1970). *Archiv. für. Ophthalmologie*, **84**, 495.

Wheelock, E. F. (1965). *Science*, **149**, 310.

Wheelock, E. F. (1966). *Proceedings of the National Academy of Sciences, USA*, **55**, 774.

Wheelock, E. F. and Larke, R. P. B. (1968). *Proceedings of the Society for Experimental Biology and Medicine*, **127**, 230.

Wheelock, E. F., Caroline, N. L. and Moore, R. D. (1971). *Journal of the National Cancer Institute*, **46**, 797.

Yamazaki, S. and Wagner, R. T. (1970). *Journal of Virology*, **5**, 220.

Youngner, J. S. and Hallum, J. V. (1969). *Virology*, **37**, 473.

Youngner, J. S., Stinebring, W. R. and Taube, S. E. (1965). *Virology*, **27**, 541.

Youngner, J. S., Thacore, H. R. and Kelly, M. E. (1972). *Journal of Virology*, **10**, 171.

Youngner, J. S., Fiengold, D. S. and Chen, J. K. (1973). *Journal of Infectious Diseases*, **128**, S227.

Subject Index

A

AH 8165, 69
Alcuronium, 65, 66, 85
Alphaxolone, 33, 39
Althesin ®, 33–40
Amyl nitrite, 93
Amylobarbitone, 3
Anaesthetics, noninhalation
  advantages, 2
  barbiturates, 2, 3–10
  buthalitone, 8, 9
  chloral hydrate, 2
  CL1848C, 43
  disadvantages, 2
  etomidate, 42
  etoxadrol, 43
  eugenols, 15–22
  G29.505, 15–16
  gamma-hydroxybutyric acid, 10
  ketamine, 11–15, 43
  methitural, 8, 9
  methohexitone, 3, 7–8
  objectives in design, 2, 41–5
  pentobarbitone, 8
  phencyclidine, 10–11
  propanidid, 16–22
  propinal, 16
  steroidal, 22–45
  testing, 41–5
  thialbarbitone, 8, 9
  thiamylal, 8, 9
  thiohexital, 8, 9
  thiopentone, 3, 4–7
  trichloroethanol, 2
Anaesthetics, steroidal
  alphadolone acetate, 33
  alphaxalone, 33, 39
  Althesin ®, 33
  clinical use
  CT1341, 31–40, 42
  discovery, 24–5
  hydroxydione, 25
  nomenclature, 22–4
  pregnane diones, 25–31, 32–40
  Saffan ®, 33

Anaesthetics, steroidal—*continued*
  solvents, 21–2, 28
  structure–activity, 26–31
  Viadril ®, 25–26
Androstane neuromuscular blockers, 60–75
Angina pectoris
  aetiology, 93
  circulatory changes in, 96–8
  exercise tests in, 95, 97
  onset mechanisms, 94
  pain thresholds, 95
  stress in, 97
  ventricular diastolic pressure, 98
Arrow poison, colombian frog, 74
1,1′-Azobis (3-methyl-2-phenyl-1*H*-imidazo(1,2-a)pyridinium) dibromide, (AH8165), 69

B

Barbiturate anaesthetics, 2, 3–10
Batrachotoxin, 74, 75
Beta-blockers in angina pectoris, 100
Buthalitone, 8, 9

C

Cardiac work, 94
Choline iodide quillaite, 74
Cona-3,5-dienine ethiodide (stercuronium), 58, 70
Conessine, 53
  dimethylconessine, 54, 56–8
Coronary artery disease, 93
Coronary dilators, 94
CT1341 (Althesin ®), 31–40
  clinical suitability, 40, 42
  clinical use, animals, 36–7
  clinical use, man, 37–9, 40
  development, 31–3
  elimination, 39–40
  formulation, 33
  metabolism, 39–40
  pharmacology, 33–36

157

Cumulative Index of Authors

Cumulative Index of Titles